Nursing Administration in the 21st Century

Nursing Administration in the 21st Century

A Self-Care Theory Approach

Sarah E. Allison
Katherine E. McLaughlin-Renpenning

SAGE Publications
International Educational and Professional Publisher
Thousand Oaks London New Delhi

For information:

SAGE Publications, Inc.
2455 Teller Road
Thousand Oaks, California 91320
E-mail: order@sagepub.com

SAGE Publications Ltd.
6 Bonhill Street
London EC2A 4PU
United Kingdom

SAGE Publications India Pvt. Ltd.
M-32 Market
Greater Kailash I
New Delhi 110048 India

Printed in the United States of America

Library of Congress Cataloging-in-Publication Data

Allison, Sarah E.
 Nursing administration in the 21st century: A self-care theory approach/ by Sarah E. Allison and Katherine E. McLaughlin-Renpenning.
  p. cm.
 Includes bibliographical references (p.   ) and index.
 ISBN 0-7619-1455-2 (cloth: acid-free paper)
 ISBN 0-7619-1456-0 (pbk.: acide-free paper)
 1. Nursing services—Administration. 2. Nursing services—Forecasting. 3. Nursing—Philosophy. I. Renpenning, Kathie McLaughlin. II. Title. III. Title: Nursing administration in the twenty-first century
 RT89.A435 1998
 362.1'73'068—ddc21   98-25382

99 00 01 02 03 04 8 7 6 5 4 3 2 1

Acquiring Editor:	Dan Ruth
Production Editor:	Astrid Virding
Editorial Assistant:	Denise Santoyo
Typesetter/Designer:	Danielle Dillahunt
Indexer:	Paul Corrington
Cover Designer:	Candice Harman

Contents

Foreword

This book is Sarah Allison's and Kathie Renpenning's response to the repeated request, "Tell us how to use a general theoretical position about nursing, specifically self-care deficit nursing theory, in the day-to-day operation of our nursing service." Both writers brought to their task a background of experiences in the study and the development of constructs of self-care deficit nursing theory, a general theory that is descriptively explanatory of nursing. They also brought to their task convictions, based on practical experiences about the value of the use of self-care deficit nursing theory in nursing practice, in the organization and operation of nursing services, and in the structuring and development of curricula for nursing educational programs.

The development of self-care deficit nursing theory during the period from 1965 to 1979 provided the basic structure for the continuing development and organization of nursing knowledge. The work of development included formulation, expression, naming, and validation of the broad conceptual elements and their relationship that were used to express the theory. The conceptual elements included self-care, self-care agency, self-care deficit, nursing agency, and nursing system. Developments during this period also included the identification of the substantive structure of each broad conceptual element named above. Substantive elements of a concept are the more narrow concepts and named features of concrete entities that constitute the structure of a broad concept such as self-care agency. The substantive elements of broad concepts identify or point to the concrete entities and relationships of nursing practice situations that nurses must know about and deal with as professionals.

The writers indicate their use of two major primary sources that address self-care deficit nursing theory and its fit within the broader framework of the nursing profession and health care services. These are the Nursing Development Conference Group's 1979 edition of *Concept Formalization in Nursing: Process and Product* and Orem's 1995 edition of *Nursing: Concepts of Practice*. Other developments of the theory expressed by the writers have some foundations in the initially developed concepts.

In the development of the book, the writers look to the future of nursing but they do not make predictions about what nursing will be. They tell us, however, what nursing can be, for nursing is something designed and produced by nurses. If nursing is the product made through the work that nurses do for and with persons under their care, then nurses' knowing what they can and should produce, why they produce it, and how to produce it in concrete life situations is critical for the continuing existence of the human health service of nursing. The content of the book should be of value to nurses and nursing students in their efforts to become experienced in thinking within a nursing frame of reference, in communicating nursing, and in practicing nursing and articulating it with broader human and health care frames of reference.

The writers use the first two chapters and Chapter 4 to discuss the settings and the features of situations where nursing is produced. Chapters 3 and 5 describe the responsibilities and work operations of nursing practitioners and nursing administrators. Chapters 6 through 12 describe specific and critical features of the work of producing nursing within health care enterprises. The content of the book is oriented to both the theoretical and the practical features of nursing and its administration.

The practical work of producing nursing or medicine or any human service is always done within a specific concrete situation of practice. For example, a surgeon at work sees and knows anatomically and physiologically the characteristics of the tissues, organs, and organ systems of the person for whom he or she is performing a surgical procedure for an agreed-on reason. As work proceeds, the surgeon makes judgments and decisions about what can and should be done in each existent but changing situation to achieve results that contribute to the human integrity of the individual for whom the surgical procedure is performed. Before and during surgery, the surgeon is aware of the health state and environmental factors that condition the patient's need for and ability to undergo surgery and the factors that condition the process of surgery. The design and plan for performance of the surgical procedure therefore not only incorporate a valid technological design of the surgical procedure but also identify and describe specific conditioning factors that affect both the patient and the surgeon's performance of the procedure.

Nurses must know the existent features of nursing practice situations where they are working. They must know the features of each situation that can be controlled or regulated and how the control or regulation can be exerted by their work for and with patients. When factors cannot be controlled or regulated, nurses act to minimize deleterious occurrences. Nursing professionals know the human and environmental factors that condition their own work and the work of their patients. They know that action based on vague impressions and generalizations is not behavior engaged in by professionals.

Sarah Allison and Kathie Renpenning have produced a book that brings to bear the nursing knowledge structured within the theoretical frame of reference of self-care deficit nursing theory on the work operations of nursing professionals and nursing administrators. These initiated developments can be taken further by interested and creative nurses. The work operations of nursing practice and nursing administration can be formalized for specific health care settings, and essential positions and units of organization can be created. Comprehensive views of populations requiring nursing, of health care enterprises, and of nursing and nurses are requisites for performance of the work of ensuring the continuing effective presence of the work of nursing in societies.

Dorothea E. Orem

Acknowledgments

First and foremost, we want to recognize Dorothea E. Orem for her significant contribution to nursing knowledge and to nursing as a practice discipline. We want to express our profound appreciation to her for sharing her conceptualizations of nursing, for her encouragement and direct assistance with this book, and most of all for her constant admonition that development of an understanding of nursing occurs in the practice setting.

To do justice in acknowledging the many nurse colleagues, friends, and family members who either directly or indirectly contributed to our thinking and work with self-care deficit nursing theory is impossible. Their help, guidance, and support are deeply appreciated. Practicing nurses who seek ways to improve care to patients and the practice of nursing provided a stimulus for this book.

We want to thank, among those who have shared their work with us, the many nurses past and present of the Mississippi Methodist Hospital and Rehabilitation Center in Jackson, Mississippi, particularly Patricia Hilkert, Irma David, Ellen Lee, and Janice McGee.

We want to thank Kathryn Long and Angela Rayborn, who have taken time to share their clinical experiences with us, helping us to validate some of the categorizations that we have derived from the theory and their usefulness to the administrator.

Dale Walker and members of the Orem Development Group and the nurses of the Vancouver Health Department, Vancouver, Canada, have made significant contributions to nursing through their work in extending the application of self-care deficit nursing theory in the community. They have generously shared their clinical experiences in several conferences and workshops providing a forum for advancing conceptualizations of nursing. We thank them for sharing the materials they have developed for client services and education of nurses.

The discussions with nurses at the Self-Care Deficit Nursing Theory Institutes sponsored by the Sinclair School of Nursing at the University of Missouri—Columbia have been invaluable. In particular, appreciation is extended to Dr. Susan Taylor, who has been instrumental in organizing those workshops and providing a vehicle for sharing thoughts, ideas, successes, and failures related to implementing theory-based nursing. Lynne Nickle has always been available for discussion and clarification as the work of the book has proceeded.

The work done under the auspices of Reuben Fernandez at Newark Beth Israel Medical Center in Newark, New Jersey, the conferences sponsored by the institution, and the contributions of the staff there as they worked to improve their practice with the assistance of nursing theory have been an impetus for writing this book and providing a guide for nursing administration.

Appreciation is extended also to the many nurses who participated in various projects of the former Center for Experimentation and Development in Nursing of the Johns Hopkins Hospital, Baltimore, Maryland, particularly the late Joan E. Backscheider.

Finally, thanks to Megan McLaughlin, who so diligently proofread versions of the manuscript at varying stages, and to Hans Renpenning, who encouraged us and put up with the confusion during the production process.

Introduction

Purpose of the Book

Ensuring the provision of nursing to individuals and patient populations now and in the future is the responsibility of professional nursing practitioners and nursing administrators. With the vast changes in the health care field, nursing leaders more than ever must have a clear vision—a mental model for nursing. Being able to conceptualize and think from a definitive nursing frame of reference provides a sound basis on which to structure and develop nursing practice in a variety of health care settings and organizations to ascertain that nursing is a visible, productive, and qualitative service. In this book, we demonstrate that a theory of nursing practice, the self-care deficit theory of nursing (Orem, 1995), facilitates developing and implementing such a mental model. A variety of conceptual structures are proposed to guide nurse administrators and nursing professionals to "think" nursing and enable them to design and develop nursing systems for a variety of patient populations. Examples of practical application are given. When nurses understand the product of nursing and the outcomes of nursing, they are in a strong position to describe the articulation of nursing with other health care professions and to communicate about nursing to the community at large. In short, the purpose of this book is to present both theoretical and practical considerations for ensuring the provision of nursing in the 21st century.

Changes in health care pose both challenges and demands for nurses and nursing as a practice discipline and a discipline of knowledge. Because nurses have diverse knowledge, skills, availability, and willingness to serve others, they are often called on and often expected to fulfill many functions, some of which are nursing and some of which are not. Maintaining the nursing focus of assisting people to manage their self-care and/or dependent care systems is essential if nursing is to survive as a profession and as an organized distinctive service to people in society. This book is not about nursing administration or nursing management per se. Other textbooks provide this information. Orem, in her foreword to this book, identifies the textbooks that set forth and explain the self-care deficit theory of nursing to which readers can refer to learn more about this theory of nursing. In this book, we show how a mental model of nursing provides a means by which nursing administration can structure and develop nursing practice and the delivery of nursing services. Examples illustrate structures and processes through which nursing administration can communicate with health care administrators, physicians, other health care members, third-party payers, and the public about patient/client requirements for nursing, nursing needs and programs, and the results to be expected from nursing. Nursing's role and contribution to health care and the benefits to be derived from nursing must be made clear to all. An adequate, comprehensive theory of nursing practice provides the means to achieve these ends.

Organization of the Book

The first chapter of this book reviews the current health care environment from which future trends must be projected and examines nursing in light of these trends. In the second chapter, the purpose of nursing and the nature of the particular service provided by nurses are described, and that service is differentiated from the services of other health care professions. In the next chapter, a view of nursing as an entity and its dimensions within the broader organizational structure is presented. A model of administration is proposed. In it, the variables of concern to nursing as revealed by self-care deficit nursing theory are utilized for forecasting nursing requirements of patient populations and projecting from these requirements the types of nurses needed to meet them and the processes that need to be in place to provide the required service. Subsequent chapters examine selected aspects of nursing administration. Overall, three major themes are explored: (a) describing nursing needs of populations; (b) specifying the knowledge and capabilities for nursing action utilizing various levels of nursing workers, with particular attention to the roles and functions of the advanced nursing practitioner and the nurse administrator; and (c) specifying administrative structures, processes, and outcomes to facilitate nursing practice. In each of these areas, models to guide thinking and practical examples are given.

Need for Nursing Theory in Nursing Administration

Without a clear theoretical basis for "thinking nursing," one reasonably might ask whether anyone, nurse or non-nurse, can fulfill the executive and managerial functions of planning and administering nursing as a service. If the administrator, whether a nurse or a non-nurse, has no formal knowledge of nursing and no basis for conceptualizing nursing, his or her approach will be strictly managerial. There will be little understanding of the product to be produced by nursing. The non-nurse manager must depend on designated nurse leaders in the organization to know and demonstrate what nursing can and should produce for the benefit of patients/clients and the organization.

Historically, management of nursing services has largely focused on the utilization of nursing resources: staffing, scheduling, assignments, and management of personnel in performing nursing activities and procedures in a humane, caring way to meet patient needs. Without a clear and consistent way to define those needs and to define and describe what nursing does and why, nursing is assumed because it is there. Too often, the contract for nursing services by health care organizations, particularly hospitals, is implied but not explicitly set forth when persons are admitted to the service. Consequently, health care providers feel free to use nonlicensed health care personnel to offer less expensive services without having a clear concept of the service nursing has to offer. Efforts to control costs associated with delivery of the nursing have resulted in using tools to measure time on task. Nursing still has not found adequate systems to accurately define nursing costs. Until recent years, no need has been felt to explain and justify nursing's particular contribution to essential operations in a health care enterprise other than to attempt to maximize the utilization of nursing resources at least cost and to coordinate nursing services with those of other health care personnel. In today's health care system, priorities have to be set and limitations in resources addressed.

How can nursing safely and effectively be provided, and to what extent can provision of nursing be ensured now and in the future? One approach to address this problem is for nursing administrators as well as nursing practitioners to have a clear focus on the domain and boundaries of nursing and the best way to utilize nursing resources to meet health goals of the populations served and goals of the organization. This requires nurses to have a clear understanding of the nature of nursing and its product—service—and involves close communication, coordination, and collaboration among nurses, other health care disciplines, administration, patients/clients, and the public.

Consideration of nursing theory as potentially useful in nursing administration began to emerge in the literature during the 1980s (Allison, McLaughlin, & Walker, 1991). In the 1990s, greater attention has been given to nursing theory in nursing administration (Fernandez & Wheeler, 1990; Huckaby, 1991; Manthey, 1991; Young & Hayne, 1988). Over the past 15 years, many health care agencies, such as hospitals, nursing homes, home health, and community health services, have adopted nursing theories such as Orem's as the basis for practice (Fawcett et al., 1990; Kerstra, Castelein, & Philipsin, 1991; Laurie-Shaw & Ives, 1988; Park, 1989; Perras & Zappacosta, 1982; Walborn, 1980; Walker, 1993). Huckaby (1991) noted the significance of nursing theory for nursing administration as a means for explaining and directing nursing practice. Barnum and Kerfoot (1995) stated that nursing theory is "the intellectual framework for patient care"; it provides "a sound basis" on which to set the "mind frame." According to them, theorizing, whether formal or informal, "is inevitable" (p. 23). Young and Hayne (1988) briefly described various valuable roles that nursing theory plays in nursing administration (pp. 67-70) but did not discuss in depth how any one theory fulfills these roles.

With the focus today on promoting people's responsibility for their own health care and a healthier lifestyle to reduce the high cost of "sick" care, the self-care deficit nursing theory is highly relevant and provides a definitive guide for designing nursing systems for patient populations for the future. The theory provides an explanation of what is required to promote and protect people's abilities for self/dependent care and to overcome self-care deficits at every stage of the health care process. Corollary to this, the nurse administrator must perceive how nursing from the self-care perspective articulates and coordinates with services provided by other health care disciplines. The nurse administrator must be visionary to foresee and conceive what can and should be done for nursing to help persons to achieve health goals, collaborate with other health care disciplines as necessary to achieve them, and reduce health care costs. Broad vision is needed to perceive and demonstrate how nursing fits into a health service organization for a particular population but also into the larger framework of health care services.

Nursing Administrative Leadership

A premise of this book is that leadership from nursing administration is essential if substantive changes in nursing practice are to be made. A nursing conceptual basis for making decisions enables development of nursing practice to achieve nursing outcomes and can provide evidence as to the particular contribution and benefits of nursing. If nursing administration or nursing management at whatever level does not take a leadership role, employed nurses will tend to be absorbed by the dominant culture—organizational, medical, or some other. An adequate conceptualization of nursing provides the basis for making decisions that support the development of nursing practice to achieve nursing outcomes and can provide evidence as to the particular contribution and benefits of nursing. Consequently, nursing administration must lead the way to demonstrate the what, how, and why of nursing by making clear nursing's purpose, focus, and boundaries—the nursing domain—and its contribution to health care. This does not preclude the collaboration of nursing in other spheres of endeavor but should make clear where nursing fits in and where it is expending effort to provide other services.

In the past, studies to advance nursing practice frequently borrowed knowledge and skills from other disciplines such as medicine. An example of this is the early work at the University of Colorado in the mid-1960s on developing the nurse practitioner role in ambulatory well-child care. This proved so successful that the role today is well established, not only in primary care for children and adults but in acute care as well. Today, this role and related functions are incorporated into both undergraduate and graduate nursing education programs. Known, validated, and standardized medical diagnostic and treatment knowledge and skills are taught to nurses and nursing students as a means of expanding the role of the nurse. But this is not nursing knowledge. It is medical knowledge. It does, however, help the nurse to understand the medical conditioning factors that establish and influence self-care demands and self-care capabilities in a nursing situation and to know more accurately when medical assistance is needed beyond what the nurse knows and can do. Advanced nursing knowledge about self-care/dependent care limitations, helping persons to meet complex self-care demands, and dealing with the factors influencing both is lacking.

Knowledge about managing self/dependent care systems needs to be developed. Knowledge borrowed from other disciplines is useful when articulated from a nursing frame of reference and can help to advance nursing knowledge.

Organizations are created and operate through the collective activities of individuals working in them toward a common purpose and having a shared vision. This requires extensive and intensive communication, cooperation, and collaboration. Nursing administration must be able to articulate and communicate the nursing perspective, how nursing can (or cannot) and does contribute to the purposes of the organization, and how nursing relates to other components in the organization. This requires the ability to clearly describe and explain nursing as a form of care required by and provided for individuals in the populations to be served, whether they are in their homes or in health care settings, based on their status as sick or healthy.

The nurse administrator's beliefs, values, concerns, and commitment to nursing, to its safe, effective delivery, and to the professional growth and development of nursing personnel are essential if the service is to be dynamic and adaptable to meet changes in health care. The leader should inspire and empower nurses to use all of their knowledge and skills and give their best for patients. Management concerns should be less in the sense of controlling relationships or the environment, asserted Morath and Manthey (1993), and more in terms of promoting the intellect and creativity of nurses. "Thinking" nursing from a theoretical perspective engages these faculties. Being able to conceptualize nursing provides a basis for developing and improving nursing practice. In this way, nursing administration becomes more than guiding and managing people. Nurse administrators or managers as leaders are responsible for examining nursing situations involving patient populations, designing and developing nursing systems of care, and planning to ensure that the essential and preferably desirable operations of nursing practice are carried out.

References

Allison, S. E., McLaughlin, K., & Walker, D. (1991). Nursing theory: A tool to put nursing back into nursing administration. *Nursing Administration Quarterly, 15*(3), 72-78.

Barnum, B. S., & Kerfoot, K. M. (1995). *The nurse as executive.* Gaithersburg, MD: Aspen.

Fawcett, J., Ellis, V., Underwood, P., et al. (1990). The effect of Orem's self-care model on nursing care in a nursing home setting. *Journal of Advanced Nursing, 15,* 659-666.

Fernandez, R. D., & Wheeler, J. L. (1990). Organizing a nursing system through theory-based practice. In G. G. Mayes, M. J. Madden, & E. Lawrenz (Eds.), *Patient delivery models* (pp. 63-83). Rockville, MD: Aspen.

Huckaby, L. M. (1991).The role of conceptual frameworks in nursing practice, administration, education, and research. *Nursing Administration Quarterly, 15*(3), 17-28.

Kerstra, A., Castelein, E., & Philipsin, H. (1991). Preventive home visits to elderly people by community nurses in the Netherlands. *Journal of Advanced Nursing, 16,* 631-637.

Laurie-Shaw, B., & Ives, S. M. (1988, March-April). Implementing Orem's self-care deficit nursing theory, part 1: Selecting a framework and planning for implementation. *Canadian Journal of Nursing Administration, 1,* 9-12.

Manthey, M. (1991). Delivery systems and practice models: A dynamic balance. *Nursing Management, 22,* 28-29.

Morath, J. M., & Manthey, M. (1993). An environment for care and service leadership: The nurse administrator's impact. *Nursing Administration Quarterly, 17*(2), 75-80.

Orem, D. E. (1995). *Nursing: Concepts of practice* (5th ed.). St. Louis, MO: Mosby Year-Book.

Park, P. B. (1989). Health care for the homeless: A self-care approach. *Clinical Nurse Specialist, 3,* 171-174.

Perras, S. T., & Zappacosta, A. R. (1982). The application of Orem's theory in promoting self-care in a peritoneal dialysis facility. *American Association of Nephrology Nurses and Technologists [AANNT] Journal, 9*(3), 37-38, 55.

Walborn, K. A. (1980). A nursing model for hospice: Primary and self-care nursing. *Nursing Clinics of North America, 15,* 205-217.

Walker, D. M. (1993). A nursing administration perspective on use of Orem's self-care deficit nursing theory. In M. Parker (Ed.), *Patterns of nursing theories in practice* (pp. 253-263). New York: National League for Nursing.

Young, L. C., & Hayne, A. N. (1988). *Nursing administration: From concepts to practice.* Philadelphia: W. B. Saunders.

CHAPTER 1

Health Care Service Organization

Trends as We Move Toward the 21st Century

A s the 21st century approaches, health care systems in Canada, the United States, and elsewhere are undergoing dramatic adjustments in response to the shrinking health care dollar, changes in population dynamics, and changes in expectations of the public about health care. This chapter gives a brief overview of some of the changes in health care organizations and services, including financing of health care. The focus is shifting from illness to wellness and integration of services along the continuum of health care. Some information is given about nurses' activities to promote and facilitate health care goals and services helping to control costs and promote quality of care. What nursing's particular contribution to health care is and can be is not always clear. This places an obligation on nursing administration to clarify the nurse's role in health care and to ensure the provision of nursing in the 21st century.

1

The Changing Structure
of the Health Care System

Although the health care systems in Canada and the United States are governed, organized, and financed differently, many of the changes that are taking place have common characteristics. Emphasis during the past decade has been on reduction in the high cost of acute hospital care. Supposedly less expensive alternatives through ambulatory care services, home health, and nursing home care have been developed and expanded.

History and Trends in Health Care

Cost containment measures began in the 1980s in the United States with the introduction of the diagnosis-related group (DRG) approach, in which reduction in the average length of stay for a diagnostic category resulted in a cost benefit for the hospital. Hospitals in Canada are also acting to reduce length of stay in inpatient settings on the basis of studies such as those done by the Health Services Utilization Research Commission (HSURC) of Saskatchewan (HSURC, 1993). These approaches to reduce the cost of inpatient acute care have resulted in the expansion and development of a variety of alternative care options, such as ambulatory day surgical care centers, day care services for elderly incapacitated patients, high-technology home care service, hospice, and use of nursing home beds for subacute care. All seek to meet community needs and integrate services for continuity of care at least cost. As a result, hospitals are downsizing, and various services are merging, consolidating, and expanding in diverse ways (Ginsberg, 1996). The challenge for the system is to develop a tracking system to determine the patient-related outcomes and the total costs across the system for the services provided.

In the United States, entrepreneurship, competition for market share, and corporatization of managed-care systems continue. Small hospitals compete by allying with ambulatory and home care facilities or are bought out by large corporations. Hospitals have been buying up practices of private physicians to ensure access to a supply of patients. Insurance companies may set up "community care networks" offering a full range of health care for a fixed price. Various facilities are acquired, thus serving to integrate and control the range of care (Weidenbaum, 1995). State and local health care corporations may expand nationally to help control costs for a mobile population but also maximize profits through economy achieved by size in purchasing power and control of competition.

In Canada, although entrepreneurship and competition for market share are not issues, similar changes in relation to mergers are occurring through the processes of regionalization of health care services. Hospitals are merging, and numbers of inpatient beds are decreasing as hospitals are closed. Outpatient services, day surgery, and home care services are expanding. Regional health authorities that are being established are being vested with powers of control for allocating resources for all health services being provided on a regional basis, including acute care, long-term care, mental health, home care, community health, diagnostic services, and ambulance services (Dorland & Davis, 1996). Although the right to health care is not incorporated into the Charter of Rights and Freedoms, among the Canadian public there is a general expectation of a right to health care (Canadian Bar Association, 1994/1996). At issue in policy making and resource allocation is the conflict between the clinician's definition of efficiency, which is to do all that is effective for the patient, and the economist's definition, which is cost based.

In both countries, vertical and horizontal integration of health care services and institutions continues to develop. Vertical integration consists of incorporating different types of health care institutions so that one feeds the other. Horizontal integration means that the corporation builds around similar institutions, typically acute care hospitals. Vertical integration will most likely replace horizontal integration in the future. There will be networking both within and outside the organization. Patient-focused designs of care under capitation arrangements will be used. All disciplines will be fluid, moving across organizational lines.

The trend in the United States is toward reliance on marketplace forces to provide safe, effective care while controlling costs and, where applicable, maximizing profits. The movement toward more involvement of the national government in health care reform currently is in abeyance. There is extensive effort to retain Medicare and Medicaid to provide for older citizens and the uninsured. Freestanding hospitals will continue to move toward integration of services, not only to control costs, but to gain or maintain access to patients and to limit competitors. Large organizations can raise capital for investment to purchase the latest technologies and expand services. The dominance of large organizations at state and local levels can have considerable political impact on a community. If marketplace forces fail to meet the public's needs and desires for assured safe and effective health care, and if health care is viewed as a "right," attempts at a political solution may again be made.

Under the 1996 national health care legislation, health care insurance is now "portable" for employees who leave one job for another. Other major players in the political arena are unions and professional organizations, such as the American Medical Association and the American Nurses Association (ANA). Unions have the power to negotiate with employers and managed-care providers for the best insurance for their members. The health professions seek their particular interests for themselves as well as society.

As organizations restructure to be cost-effective, consolidation may take the form of "downsizing," especially cutting beds in acute care facilities, integrating services, and "flattening" the layer of management to bring managers closer to the operational level and make them more responsive to it. In nursing, "shared governance," in which nurses participate in decisions affecting them and their work, is a form of unification within a service.

In the United States, control of the market by third-party payers, both government and private insurance, portends a short life for small independent health care agencies and institutions. Although the controlling mechanisms are different, the result is the same. Small independent health care agencies are becoming a thing of the past in Canada also. Efforts to consolidate are one means of controlling administrative costs for the private practice of doctors and intermediaries. These costs are estimated to run from about 16% to 30% of the health care dollar per year (Frey, 1995, Appendix). The growth in the ratio of physicians to the general population, particularly specialists, is estimated to be about 75% of health system costs (Ginsberg, 1996). Management control measures employed include use of primary care physicians to control referrals to specialists; case managers to monitor, direct, and control use of resources; and less expensive health care providers—nurse practitioners, nurse midwives, and physician assistants—to provide care. In the United States, employers and unions as major purchasers of health care seek to control costs by choosing plans that endeavor to keep patients out of expensive hospitals and provide a full range of care services less expensively.

■ Managed Care

With prospective payment systems, *managed care* is a term that has a variety of meanings. Principally, the idea is to seek quality of care in a cost-effective manner through some form of control mechanism, such as case management. The case manager may be a social worker, a nurse, a physician, or some other person knowledgeable about health care. Frequently, nurses make excellent case managers because of their medical and nursing knowledge, especially when they have some community health background. Case management is used by third-party payers and hospitals to help control costs in use of services and yet ensure safe, effective provision of care. According to Cohen and Cesta (1997), managed care is a delivery system for cost-effective patient outcomes that usually is unit based—at the bedside. Case management may also entail direct accountability and responsibility for the delivery of care for a DRG, regardless of geographic location in the hospital. Managed care seeks to ensure consistency in care while controlling costs throughout a hospital stay. Predetermined care maps or protocols delineate common activities to be performed and outcomes to be anticipated for particular types of patients over a defined period of time during the course of stay and possibly beyond.

According to Moningham and Scott (1997), there are three aspects of managed care: (a) the fiscal aspects of cost containment, (b) care management for quality of care and cost containment, and (c) nursing case management, which includes various case management and care activities for patient problems and needs in the community. In future planning for delivery of health care services, designs of care systems will not be limited to one setting but will take into consideration the whole trajectory of health care. In this, nursing should play a leading role. In the majority of cases, nursing is the primary type of health care service needed because of persons' dependence in performing self-care over a continuing period of time.

Financing of Health Care in the United States

How will health care in the United States be financed and provided in the future? Currently, the United States outspends all other countries on health care: 40% of the gross domestic product (GDP) is spent on the health care system (Ginsberg, 1996). The United States and South Africa are the only nations without national health insurance systems (Shemhusen, 1995). The U.S. public tends to be antigovernment in terms of control of health care, yet desirous of some form of protection for all. In light of these factors, Ginsberg (1996) suggested that there will be a "renewed confrontation with health care reform" sometime in the future (p. 154).

Efforts at welfare reform in the United States have just begun with the 1996 legislation, the impact of which remains to be seen. The thrust toward alleviating dependency on the government for subsistence is an attempt to force people to become self-supporting and to prevent them from being reliant for generations on the government for support. Not all employers provide for health care. To survive, many new workers, former welfare recipients, and the unemployed will continue to require health care and some means to pay for it. In the past, this was done by hospitals through cost shifting or subsidization to offset the cost of charity care. Those who could pay, private patients, helped to provide for the nonpaying patients. Government support will continue to be needed for this purpose. In the future, decisions about how best to spend available monies will reside with state and local governments, where local needs and potentials are best understood. Difficulties may arise, however, in the poorer, less populous states, where the tax base is more limited unless nationally funded grants are provided.

Under past payment systems, insurance frequently paid the bills, and the consumer did not have to worry about personally paying for health care. Thus, the consumer was not as concerned about the cost of health care. Today, the high cost of health care is a concern to all and has been highly politicized. Frequently, as individuals or in groups, consumers select a managed-care plan provider of health care. Consequently, insurers are increasingly concerned, not only about general health outcomes and costs, but about patient/client satisfaction with the care provided. In a competitive environment, clients may choose another managed-care provider if they are not satisfied with the quality and amount of care provided under a given plan. As a result, and with the trend toward greater emphasis on responsibility for one's own personal health care, patients now are more likely to be recognized as partners in the care process. Difficulty may occur, however, when a patient chooses to have a physician or service that is not a part of his or her health care plan. This problem of choice may arise when a particularly complex or unique health care problem requires a particular specialist or health care service not in the plan. The patient may then have to pay for the service personally or negotiate for the care with the plan and provider. The loss of freedom of choice of health care providers has already been a source of dissatisfaction for some.

Managed-care systems may be organized as health maintenance organizations, preferred provider organizations, physician-hospital organizations, or other arrangements. Payment to hospitals and physicians after care has been provided (retrospective payment) is a thing of the past. Use of a personal physician on a fee-for-service basis becomes limited to those who are not members of prepaid insurance plans and can afford to pay for the service. One cost containment method projected for the future is prospective payment, the setting of fees for services in advance, with a fixed amount allotted per DRG or a discount arrangement between hospital and payer. Capitation is being advocated by some as a means to control costs. It is a set amount of money allocated per individual for all health care provided, no matter what the cost. Ginsberg (1996) noted, however, that capitation shifts the risk from the managed-care provider to the hospital and physician. The major concern of the public is to be assured of safe, effective care at a reasonable cost and to retain decision-making power about the care process. If or when dissatisfaction with the availability of or access to desired care and quality of care occurs, there again may well be a shift in how health care is provided and paid for. Some evidence of this is beginning to be seen in situations in which profits and/or cost controls appear to take precedence over patient needs, desires, and quality of care.

Financing of Health Care in Canada

The majority of health care services in Canada are financed one way or another through tax dollars. Both the federal and the provincial governments have a role in financing of health care, and now that regionalization of health care services has been implemented or endorsed by most provinces in Canada, sorting out the roles, responsibilities, and decision-making powers of the federal, provincial, and regional authorities and local boards has become more complex and in many ways more politicized. The provinces are responsible for the delivery of health care, but this cannot be accomplished without input from the federal government. Fortier (1996), in describing the role of the federal government, pointed out that federal involvement is related to three powers vested in that government:

1. *Criminal law,* which is the basis for such legislation as the Narcotics Control Act and the Food and Drug Act. These statutes affect the health of persons and health care services delivery.
2. *Spending power,* which includes the power to levy taxes and distribute funds. Through distribution of funds, the federal government has tried to even out monetary discrepancies between rich and poor provinces, enabling all Canadians to benefit equally from social programs such as pensions and health services.
3. *Peace, order, and good government,* which have been the basis for addressing areas of national concern, including maintaining countrywide standards in areas such as health.

The federal government is also responsible directly for delivery of services to First Nations people on reserves, Correctional Services, members of the armed forces and veterans, and, partially, the Royal Canadian Mounted Police. Several branches of government set national standards: Health Canada regulates drugs and medical devices, Fisheries and Oceans monitors safety of fish and seafood purchased by consumers, and Environment Canada monitors land, air, and water quality. The federal government supports the health care system through the Canada Health Act, federal-provincial transfer payments, and research funding. The federal government also exercises responsibility in relation to health promotion, illness prevention, and education.

At present, there is an uneasy feeling in Canada about the future of the health care system, the extent of the control that the federal government will continue to exercise or not exercise, and the possible erosion of the universal health care system, which has come to be perceived as a fundamental value by many Canadians. This uneasy feeling has come about as a result of changes proposed in the transfer of funds to the provinces. The transfer of funds began after the Second World War and has continued in various forms, such as grants, cost sharing, and block transfers. Some of these funds were specifically targeted, some had attached conditions, and others could be allocated as provinces wished. In 1995, the federal government announced the Canada Health and Social Transfer Program, which would combine social and health transfers to the provinces, leaving the provinces free to determine resource allocation. The fear is that with this change in transfer payments the federal government will lose its ability to maintain the principles of the Canada Health Act—the assurance of a universal, accessible, comprehensive, portable, and publicly funded health care system.

At the provincial level, there has been widespread support for the development of regionalized systems, some with elected boards and some with appointed boards. Essentially, the regional authorities are taking over administration of health care services financed by the provincial governments. Fraser (1996) outlined the functions in relation to health care service delivery as planning, resource allocation, policy development, standard setting, coordination, evaluation, and delivery, with responsibility for these functions resting either at the provincial level or at the level of the regional authority. He suggested that there could be a "marriage of policy and operational functions," with the regional authority being accountable and liable for design and provision of care to the region. One outcome of this marriage could be that regional authorities would be held liable for inadequate system design and negligent provision of care. This has implications for the process of ensuring safe, effective provision of specific health care services (a topic dealt with in the following chapters).

Nursing Role Concerning Costs
and Quality of Care

It is recognized that efforts to control costs can affect the quality of patient care. In 1996, the *American Journal of Nursing* conducted an opinion survey of over 7,000 nurses about the effects of downsizing, restructuring, and use of unlicensed personnel on patient care. Some of its findings were that fewer nurses are taking care of more patients, have less time for all aspects of care to patients, have more responsibilities, and are being cross-trained to care for a variety of patients. Findings suggest less continuity of care, an increase in hospital readmission of patients, the perception of a decrease in the quality of care, especially in subacute care facilities, an increase in work-related injuries, and other concerns (Shindul-Rothschild, Berry, & Long-Middleton, 1996).

Nursing Activities in the United States

The ANA has actively lobbied Congress regarding health matters of concern to nursing and in relation to the public welfare of the people. Similarly, state districts monitor and lobby state legislatures. The ANA and other professional nursing groups seek media attention on health issues and participate in a variety of activities to raise public awareness of potential problem areas. For example, in 1998 in Massachusetts, a number of nurses and physicians joined together to protest for-profit managed-care organizations that might tend to maximize profits over quality of care. They expressed their concerns to the news media by holding a "Boston tea party" and throwing the annual reports of these organizations into the Boston harbor ("Mass. Nurses," 1998). In the United States, nurses become involved in promoting health and well-being for the less advantaged through volunteer work (e.g., in street clinics), through participating in new delivery systems of health care undertaken by various public and private organizations, and through conducting studies to demonstrate the benefits and inadequacies of care on patient outcomes (Blegen, Goode, & Reed, 1998). Similarly, in Canada, the Saskatchewan Union of Nurses undertook extensive data gathering in an effort to determine the public's perception of health care services following institution of regional health boards, consolidation of services, and downsizing.

Both clinical and financial research are needed to definitively evaluate the impact of the various economic moves on the quality of care. Currently, emphasis is being placed on continuous quality improvement and monitoring of various systems for providing care. Mohr and Mahon (1996) warned of the "dirty hands" potential in large health care provider systems, where the profit motive may encourage unethical or illegal activities. Employees may be intimidated not to tell for fear of job loss in a tight market. The health care worker must be committed to safe care and control of costs but also must be aware of potential abuses and failures to provide needed care.

Various control and monitoring mechanisms have been used in the past, such as certificates of need, peer review, utilization review to determine appropriate utilization of resources, and quality assessment programs. Some agencies have established physician profiles to assess excess or misuse of resources. Attempts at medical malpractice reform seek to reduce the high cost of tort liability. Doctors may order tests not because of apparent clinical need but as protection in case some unforeseen finding results in legal action.

A current strategy to control costs is the use of guidelines, critical paths, or care maps as standardized care protocols to be followed during various phases in the care process for selected common DRGs. These serve both clinical and cost containment purposes. Nursing care indicators for nursing outcomes and nursing actions required may or may not be clearly delineated in these protocols. A national nursing study found that existing outcome studies did not typically focus on isolating the contribution of nursing when measuring the quality of care and recommended that future studies do this (Wunderlich, Sloan, & Davis, 1996). Nursing's contribution to health care will remain obscure if it is not clearly evident in these protocols, in nursing documentation, and through other means.

McCloskey et al. (1996) reviewed four management innovations that had been predicted to enhance service and contain costs: nurse extenders, hospital-based case management, nursing shared governance, and product-line management. They found that systematic evaluation strategies for designing and delivering effective and efficient management of nursing services were lacking. They contended that research related to these innovations is plagued with several difficulties:

1. Complex innovations lack clear definitions.
2. Innovations are often implemented with other changes, making it difficult to isolate the effect.
3. The group level of measurement makes it difficult to obtain large samples.
4. The intervening variables are not often identified, controlled for, or measured.
5. The effects on staff and patients tend to be ignored. (p. 13)

Nursing Activities in Canada

In Canada, there is increasing emphasis on health promotion, with a major research undertaking being funded across Canada by National Health and Welfare and the Social Sciences and Humanities Research Council. Six centers for health promotion research were established in 1993 under a 5-year national program. These centers are exploring individual and societal issues affecting people's health and were charged with developing new approaches to promote healthy living and working conditions (J. Feather, personal communication, 1993). There also is the potential for a paradigm shift away from the predominant medical model for health care delivery. Mhatre and Deber (1992) analyzed policy options of provincial reports that were the result of activities occurring in response to Health Minister Jake Epp's (1986) document *Achieving Health for All* and the release of the Ottawa Charter for Health Promotion ("Ottawa Charter," 1986), two documents that set the stage for establishment of provincial advisory committees, task forces, and commissions focusing on health care reform. Commonly recurring themes were use of a broader definition of health; intersectoral planning; emphasis on health promotion and disease prevention, with a partial rejection of the medical model; a shift from institutional to community-based care; and efforts to increase public participation, particularly in planning and developing regional authorities. On the provincial level, activities such as the establishment in Saskatchewan of the Population Health and Evaluation Research Unit (HSURC, 1997), a partnership of the provincial government, the universities, the health district system of the Medical Research Council of Canada, and HSURC, holds promise for some research-based activities and decision making in health care planning.

The Canadian Nurses Association (CNA) has been actively promoting the principles of primary health care—health promotion, public participation, intersectoral and interdisciplinary collaboration, accessibility, and appropriate technology—through development of policy statements (CNA, 1988, 1989a, 1991). The implementation of these strategies is evidenced in briefs and publications of the CNA (1989b, 1990, 1993a, 1993b). The provincial nursing associations also have been actively involved in supporting primary health care activities. Rodger and Gallagher (1995) listed projects organized by provincial nurses' associations that are related to health promotion. A few of these are

- A pilot project of a community-based health center undertaken by the Association of Nurses of Prince Edward Island

- ※ A health education in schools program undertaken by the Registered Nurses Association of British Columbia
- ※ The Northwest Territories Ranklin Inlet Project
- ※ Health promotion projects in Quebec
- ※ 11 community forums in Saskatchewan

In addition, British Columbia instituted a nurse-managed clinic, and Saskatchewan piloted a project that fostered an expanded role for nurses in a rural clinic. Manitoba is creating community nurses' resource centers. The government of Alberta is supporting the Increased Direct Access to Nursing Services project of the nurses' association. Public participation has been augmented not only through the lobbying efforts of the nurses' associations but also by encouragement of community members to attend and present issues at district health board meetings and to participate in commissions related to health care reform and by lobbying actions of such groups as the Health Action Lobby ("HEAL on the Move," 1991).

As nursing becomes more and more involved in the health care planning process and delivery of expanded services, the role of nursing theory in providing direction for the design and delivery of nursing services becomes more and more significant. The role of nursing theory in these processes is the major theme of this book.

Changing Requirements for Job-Related Skills

In the future, with mergers, consolidation, and redesign of health care systems, ensuring continuity of care will require continuity of information, a decrease in paperwork, and a need for protection of confidentiality of patient information. Electronic information systems are becoming more and more necessary. Health care workers must become computer literate, not only to operate the equipment, but to ensure that systems are designed that meet their information needs.

Emphasis will be on interdisciplinary approaches to health care and close collaboration between health care disciplines. Skills of negotiation and cooperation are essential. Interdependence among professionals broadens the base of decision making and requires autonomy in the mode of operations as new models for delivery of care are developed. Nurses must be clear about their role and function as nurses and about what nursing has to offer to patient welfare if they are to contribute effectively to the health team. Nursing must not simply take on tasks of others without understanding the implications for nursing and for increasing nursing effectiveness.

The reduction in acute care hospital beds means that nurses on inpatient services must be cross-trained, not only to work with different patient populations in a hospital, but perhaps to work in ambulatory and home health settings as well. Rodger and Gallagher (1995) reported that the majority of university nursing education programs have significantly increased their primary health care content, including courses on community development, community assessment, and community health practice with populations at the undergraduate level and on community health streams at the graduate level. Working in the community requires that nurses develop knowledge and skills such as empowerment strategies (Duncan, 1996), collaborative skills (Chalmers & Bramadat, 1996), negotiation, political strategies, and participatory research. They will also have to develop skill in using "data from direct client work to inform the community of needs and problems" (Chalmers & Bramadat, 1996, p. 724). In the following chapters of this book, we will demonstrate how the use of nursing theory can facilitate that process. Chapter 4's discussion on describing populations from a nursing perspective, Appendix 4A's identification of the variables of concern to nursing, and Chapter 7's discussion of the nursing component of the clinical communication system are all particularly pertinent to the process.

With the move to provide services for individuals and populations across the age span and across the continuum of agencies, designing, developing, and utilizing an appropriate communication system that accommodates storage and rapid retrieval of data from a variety of sites and tracking of individuals and populations become important. Nurses must develop skills that enable them to participate with persons familiar with information management strategies and computer systems design in the development of such systems. As described in Chapter 7, a nursing practice theory can facilitate this process. Many nurses in the workforce today have limited knowledge of and experience with nursing theories. This deficiency must be corrected if adequate information systems for nursing purposes are to be developed and if nursing is to be a full partner in the development of data banks and information-processing systems (Bliss-Holtz, Taylor, & McLaughlin, 1992; Hays, Norris, Martin, & Androwich, 1994).

Unification of Services

Unification of health care services occurs on many levels. Integration of services at the organizational level is taking place through the continuum of care as hospitals, ambulatory care services, home health, and nursing home organizations coalesce. At the multidisciplinary level, health care disciplines in matrix organizations plan and implement health care together. Clinical care pathways or care maps are developed as standard protocols for the processes and outcomes of care by DRG, thus serving both clinical and financial control purposes. Insurers, both government and private, cooperate with these programs and organizations to achieve cost-effective results from the payers' perspective. Nursing service organizational structures are also being redesigned to give nurses more responsibility, accountability, autonomy, and authority, not only over nursing, but over coordination of nursing with the services of other health professions. Emphasis today is on multidisciplinary teamwork at the patient operational level. Physicians, nurses, and other health care disciplines are collaborating, making decisions about care, and coordinating their efforts on patients' behalf. The nurse case manager has emerged as a key figure in seeking unification of services through effective utilization of resources for both clinical and financial purposes. Through the foregoing, unification of health care services is taking place on many levels in both Canada and the United States.

In the United States, one concern has been the overabundance of physician specialists and the lack of sufficient primary care physicians. Medical schools are seeking to rectify this inadequacy. In Canada, medical education has changed considerably in the past few years, with students being required to choose family practice or a specialty much earlier in the course of their education. This change is too recent for the outcome to be evaluated. A problem common to both countries has been the lack of sufficient physicians in rural, less populated, and less affluent areas. In Canada, there has been a change in how health care is provided as small rural hospitals are systematically being closed. Expanded roles for nursing, use of nonphysician providers, computer interactive medical consultations, and air transportation to medical centers are some means of compensating for the lack of physicians and health care facilities.

From the clinician's point of view, unification of services requires an alteration in perspective as to where a particular discipline may overlap with another and where there may be gaps to be filled by someone. This takes systems thinking and deliberate planning concerning the contribution of each discipline to the total welfare of the patients to be served. It also demands a clear focus and understanding of one's own discipline to identify how best to contribute, where to coordinate and collaborate, and what "trade-offs" can be made for more effective functioning—a theme that is constantly referred to in this book. Manion and Watson (1995) warned that deemphasizing the uniqueness of nursing as a discipline may be "potentially destructive" in the long run (p. 255). They pointed out that the very uniqueness of each person and profession on a team is what makes the team effective. Differences must be recognized and valued for what each contributes to the whole. Multidisciplinary and interdisciplinary teams must thoroughly examine and identify ways in which to function more effectively and efficiently, given the organization, the characteristics of the patients, and the situation. The major challenge to both health care providers and the system of health care is to rethink their current mode of operation and functioning to meet the changes that are occurring and will continue to occur.

Need to Recognize and Plan for the Production of Specific Health Care Services

In the current literature, there is much emphasis on the need for interdisciplinary cooperation and cross-training to achieve the goals of vertical and horizontal integration and cost-effective service delivery. There is merit in both of these trends. Nurses are in an ideal position to facilitate interdisciplinary cooperation in the interests of achieving integration because they have more hours of contact with the users of the health care system across the life span than any other health care professionals and also are frequently the coordinators of services. Historically, though not being the recipients of formalized cross-training, nurses have performed tasks associated with medicine, physiotherapy, occupational therapy, social work, dietetics, and pharmacy when these professional services are not available on a 24-hour, 7-day-a-week basis, and they continue to do so. Often, this has been to the detriment of the nursing component. Planning specifically for the production of nursing is essential to ensuring that the service is provided.

Planning for the production of the service includes naming the service, identifying the outcomes of provision of the service, establishing appropriate budget allocation, providing personnel, and establishing processes and procedures related to production. The product of nursing is a system of actions and interactions between the patient/client, his or her caregivers, and the nurse to meet the goals of the patient/client's health-related self-care. The outcome of this activity is promotion of life, health, well-being, and development through meeting the therapeutic self-care demand and regulating self-care agency. In other words, the role of the nurse is to help the patient and family to establish and enact a health-related self-management system. Patients/clients may require

TABLE 1.1 Complementary Relationships of Nursing to Other Disciplines

Discipline and Associated Role/Goal	Nursing
Physician—Recognize presence of threats to health and establish treatment/prevention regime.	Assist individuals to incorporate therapy into system of daily living and to develop skills required for therapeutic regime. Provide care if necessary. Recognize need for and refer to physicians.
Physiotherapy—Establish/supervise an appropriate exercise program.	Assist individuals to incorporate exercise program into overall system of daily living. Recognize need for and refer to physiotherapist.
Social Worker—Assess need and assist with access to community resources.	Incorporate assistance from community resources into systems of daily living. Recognize need for and refer to social worker.
Family Therapist—Assess, facilitate, and provide counseling in relation to family functioning.	Assess, facilitate, and counsel regarding relationship between family functioning and self-care.

only nursing or they may require the services of other disciplines. Table 1.1 illustrates the complementary relationships of nursing to other disciplines.

It is the responsibility of nursing to plan for the production of its services. In a recent study of current trends in the health care service in Canada, the researchers found that board members of health care authorities were least pleased with their orientation to assessing health care needs and that their activities were most related to setting priorities, ensuring effectiveness and efficiency of services, and allocating funds and least related to production of services. In addition, information on population needs was available for decision making less often than information on service costs; hence, decisions were made by looking at budgets rather than health needs (Lomas, Veenstra, & Woods, 1997).

Undoubtedly, one of the difficulties that has faced nursing and that continues to be an issue is the number of nurses with administration responsibilities who would ordinarily be responsible for planning for the production of nursing but who have little or no background in nursing theory and who are unable to describe nursing and its contribution as other than a series of tasks, many of which have their origin in the activities of other disciplines.

**Ensuring the Provision of Nursing:
Theoretical and Practical Considerations**

This topic is dealt with in detail in subsequent chapters and is addressed only briefly here. To ensure the provision of nursing within a multidisciplinary health care enterprise, there must be a clear definition of what is meant by nursing and what nursing can and does accomplish. For the past 100 years, much of nursing has taken place under the control of the health care delivery system. It has not been under the control of the profession, as has medicine or other health professions. The strategies employed by nurses to accomplish their work frequently have been controlled or prescribed by the enterprise through such organizational tools as policy and procedure manuals, standard care plans, and now managed-care plans. Within this constraining environment, individual nurses have developed strategies that "have worked," so they have continued to use them, sometimes sharing these strategies with others but frequently keeping them to themselves.

With the increase in university-prepared nurses and graduate education, there has been a corresponding increase in research related to nursing. In some of this research, investigators ask nursing questions and investigate from a nursing perspective. Much of the research is within the theoretical frameworks of other disciplines, so that questions are structured and investigated from another discipline's perspective. In part, this is because the graduate education of nurses has taken place outside of nursing—in education, administration, physiology, and so on. Many of the nurses who have taken their advanced education have little knowledge of nursing theory and little understanding of the contribution that nursing theory can make to nursing practice, administration, and research. A senior nursing administrator at a nursing theory conference complained about the language used by theorists to describe the phenomena with which they were concerned. Her graduate degree was in business administration, and her comment was, "I can't understand what those people are talking about. I have a better understanding of the terms associated with accounting than I do of the terms they are using to describe nursing." The lack of senior nursing personnel with advanced degrees in nursing is preventing the nursing profession from making the contribution that it should be making within the interdisciplinary environment in the health care field today. Moreover, few, if any, nursing administration textbooks fully address the utility of nursing theory for developing nursing practice and organization for that practice.

Nursing is a practice discipline with a theoretical aspect and a practical aspect. The knowledge base of the practical component necessarily develops within the practice arena, with direction from the theoretical component. If the nursing theorists have little access to or experience with the practice arena and the practitioners have no association with the theoretical component, the development of practical knowledge is limited, fragmented, and not disseminated among the practitioners as it should be. Each health care enterprise, through the policies that it implements and the nature of the practice environment afforded nursing (either restrictive or creative), plays a major role in the development or lack of development of the knowledge base of nursing.

Research is foundational to the development of the knowledge base of nursing and ultimately to the delivery and development of the nursing component of quality health care. This research must take place in the health care enterprise, for that is where the bulk of the clinical experiences of the nurse occurs. At present, there is very little interest within the "work" environment to fund such activity. Yet it is essential to the efficient and effective delivery of nursing services. Medicine has advanced to the stage it has by case-by-case study of therapeutic strategies, carefully constructed research projects comparing those strategies, and dissemination of that information to the practitioners. Nursing is only beginning to embark on this course of action through the impetus of such organizations as Sigma Theta Tau, which has specifically listed the dissemination of nursing knowledge as one of its objectives; the establishment of the Center for Nursing Research at the National Institutes of Health; the establishment of chairs for nursing research at universities; the increase in the number of doctoral programs; and the setting of the goal of entry to practice as a baccalaureate degree. Each health care enterprise providing nursing services has a responsibility not only to contribute to the knowledge base of the service called nursing but not to prevent development of that knowledge base by denigrating nursing education and nursing research or by denying that it has a responsibility in relation to nursing knowledge development.

Summary

With constant changes in society and health care organizations, increasing costs of health care, and increasing efforts to contain those costs, nursing, other health care professions, and the public are all profoundly affected. Major concerns in both the United States and Canada are to have assurance of availability and access to health care and to quality of care. Nursing, as the largest workforce in health care, has a major role to play in providing health care. The particular contribution of nursing to health care and benefits to be derived from nursing must be made clear. This is not evident in the review of the changes that are occurring and the nursing activities being performed for the benefit of nursing as a profession and for patient welfare. Nursing administration has the responsibility to assume leadership in designing, planning, and ensuring the provision of nursing as a distinctive beneficial service to patient/client populations now and in the future.

References

Blegen, M. A., Goode, C. J., & Reed, L. (1998). Nurse staffing and patient outcomes. *Nursing Research, 47*(1), 43-50.

Bliss-Holtz, J., Taylor, S., & McLaughlin, K. (1992). Nursing theory as a base for computerized nursing information system. *Nursing Science Quarterly, 5,* 124-128.

Canadian Bar Association. (1996). What's law got to do with it? Health reform in Canada. In J. L. Dorland & S. M. Davis (Eds.), *How many roads: Regionalization and decentralization in health care.* Kingston, Ontario: Queen's University, School of Policy Studies. (Original work published 1994)

Canadian Nurses Association. (1988). *Health for all Canadians: A call for health care reform.* Ottawa: Author.

Canadian Nurses Association. (1989a). *Health care reform for seniors.* Ottawa: Author.

Canadian Nurses Association. (1989b). *Submission to the Standing Committee of the House of Commons on Health and Welfare, Social Affairs, Seniors and the Status of Women: Select issues in health care delivery.* Ottawa: Author.

Canadian Nurses Association. (1990). *New reproductive technologies: Accessible, appropriate, participative. Brief for the Royal Commission on New Reproductive Technologies.* Ottawa: Author.

Canadian Nurses Association. (1991). *Mental health care reform: A discussion paper of mental health care.* Ottawa: Author.

Canadian Nurses Association. (1993a). *Nurses know, nurses can: An election handbook.* Ottawa: Author.

Canadian Nurses Association. (1993b). *Nurses make the difference: A brief on cost effective nursing alternatives.* Ottawa: Author.

Chalmers, K. I., & Bramadat, I. J. (1996). Community development: Theoretical and practical issues for community health nursing in Canada. *Journal of Advanced Nursing, 24,* 719-726.

Cohen, E. L., & Cesta, T. G. (1997). *Nursing case management: From concept to evaluation* (2nd ed.). St. Louis: C. V. Mosby.

Dorland, J. L., & Davis, S. M. (1996). Introduction: Regionalization as health care reform. In J. L. Dorland & S. M. Davis (Eds.), *How many roads: Regionalization and decentralization in health care* (pp. 3-7). Kingston, Ontario: Queen's University, School of Policy Studies.

Duncan, S. M. (1996). Empowerment strategies in nursing: A foundation for population-focussed clinical studies. *Public Health Nursing, 5,* 311-317.

Epp, J. (1986). *Achieving health for all: A framework for health promotion.* Ottawa: Minister of Supply and Services.

Fortier, M. (1996). The evolving federal role in health care. In J. L. Dorland & S. M. Davis (Eds.), *How many roads: Regionalization and decentralization in health care* (pp. 15-23). Kingston, Ontario: Queens University, School of Policy Studies.

Fraser, R. (1996). Accountability and regionalization. In J. L. Dorland & S. M. Davis (Eds.), *How many roads: Regionalization and decentralization in health care* (pp. 33-50). Kingston, Ontario: Queens University, School of Policy Studies.

Frey, W. R. (Ed.). (1995). *Cross national perspectives on health care reform.* Buffalo, NY: William S. Heent.

Ginsberg, E. (1996). *Tomorrow's hospital: A look to the twenty-first century.* New Haven, CT: Yale University Press.

Hays, B. J., Norris, J., Martin, K. S., & Androwich, I. (1994). Informatics issues for nursing's future. *Advances in Nursing Science, 16*(4), 71-78.

HEAL on the move. (1991). *CNA Today, 1*(3), 1-2.

Health Services Utilization and Research Commission. (1993). *Barriers to community care.* Saskatoon, Saskatchewan: Author.

Health Services Utilization and Research Commission. (1997, Summer). New population health research unit promises benefits for many sectors. *A Closer Look,* p. 1.

Lomas, J., Veenstra, G., & Woods, J. (1997). Devolving authority for health care in Canada's provinces: 2. Backgrounds, resources and activities of board members. *Canadian Medical Association Journal, 156,* 513-520.

Manion, J., & Watson, P. M. (1995). Developing team-based patient care through re-engineering. In S. M. Blancett & D. I. Flarey (Eds.), *Reengineering nursing and health care.* Gaithersburg, MD: Aspen.

Mass. nurses, docs spark health care revolution. (1998). *American Nurse, 30*(1), 6.

McCloskey, J. C., Maas, M. L., Huber, D. G., Kasparek, A., Specht, J. P., Ramler, C. L. Watson, C., Blegen, M. A., Delaney, C., Ellerbe, S., Etscheidt, C., Gongawera, C., Johnson, M. R., Kelly, K. C., Mehmert, P., & Clougherty, J. (1996). Nursing management innovations: A need for systematic evaluation. In K. C. Kelly & M. L. Maas (Eds.), *Outcomes of effective management practice* (pp. 3-19). Thousand Oaks, CA: Sage.

Mhatre, S. L., & Deber, R. (1992). From equal access to health care to equitable access to health: Review of Canadian provincial commissions and reports. *International Journal of Health Services, 22,* 645-668.

Mohr, W. K., & Mahon, M. M. (1996). "Dirty hands": The underside of marketplace health care. *Advances in Nursing Science, 19,* 28-37.

Moningham, L., & Scott, C. B. (1997). A model emerges for the community-based nurse care management of older adults. *Nursing and Health Care Perspective on Community, 18*(2), 68-73.

Ottawa Charter for Health Promotion. (1986). *Canadian Journal of Public Health, 77,* 425-430.

Rodger, G. L., & Gallagher, S. M. (1995). The move toward primary health care in Canada: Community health nursing from 1985 to 1995. In M. J. Stewart (Ed.), *Community nursing: Promoting Canadians' health.* Toronto: W. B. Saunders.

Shemhusen, J. (1995). U.S. health care reform: Sold out to the highest bidder. In W. R. Frey (Ed.), *Cross national perspectives on health care reform.* Buffalo, NY: William S. Heent.

Shindul-Rothschild, J., Berry, D., & Long-Middleton, E. (1996). Where have all the nurses gone? Final results of our patient care survey. *American Journal of Nursing, 96*(11), 25-39.

Weidenbaum, M. (1995). A new look at health care reform. In W. R. Frey (Ed.), *Cross national perspectives on health care reform.* Buffalo, NY: William S. Heent.

Wunderlich, G. S., Sloan, F. A., & Davis, C. K. (1996). *Nursing staff in hospitals and nursing homes: Is it adequate?* Washington, DC: Institute of Medicine.

The Domain of Nursing

Persons on a day-to-day basis are responsible for and manage their own health care. When specialized knowledge, skills, and technologies are needed, services of health care professionals are sought. Health care enterprises exist to meet the needs of the community, and administrators responsible for providing these services collaborate with health care professionals and funding sources to ensure that quality of care and cost-effective services are provided. Planning and development of health care programs requires knowledge of the community's needs; the sociocultural, economic, and political factors influencing health and health care services; and the general personal characteristics and capabilities of the target population.

In this chapter, the value of knowing the focus or proper object of each health care discipline is discussed, and models are presented illustrating the role and responsibilities of patients/clients and their caregivers in managing health-related matters. The articulation between these models and the particular domain and responsibilities of nursing as expressed in self-care deficit nursing theory is described. A model illustrating interdisciplinary relationships is also presented.

The Value of a Mental Model

The nature of the services offered by a health care enterprise is influenced by the vision or mental model that the developers have of the service to be produced.

Senge (1990) described mental models as "the medium through which we and the world interact" (pp. xi-xv). They are "the deeply ingrained assumptions, generalizations, even pictures or images that influence how we understand the world and how we take action. We may or may not be consciously aware of them, but we act upon them" (p. 8).

Senge (1990) advocated creating meaning and setting a perspective through a mental model as a means for focusing on the continued improvement of a system or an organization. He stated that organizations ultimately work the way they do because of how they think and act. Although the trend in today's health care organization is to redesign external structures, they must address the "internal structures of our mental model" because "we are our mental models" (p. xv).

The problem is to obtain the congruence of our mental model of the health care service to be delivered—in this case, nursing— with the models of others in the health care enterprise or profession. This requires building what Senge (1990) called the "shared vision"—a shared picture of the future that we seek to create" (p. 9). To do this, personal mastery, team learning, and systems thinking are required. Personal mastery depends on continuous learning to perceive how our actions affect the world. Team learning requires suspension of previous assumptions and entering into genuine *thinking* together with others. This, in turn, necessitates systems thinking if we are to create a better future. It means seeing things as "wholes," seeing interrelationships rather than things, and seeing patterns of change. Senge (1990) called systems thinking "the fifth discipline—shifting the mind from seeing parts to wholes. People are active participants in shaping reality, creating the future, not just reacting to events" (p. 64).

Systems thinking requires a mental model, "for without it the power is lost" (Senge, 1990, p. 209). A shared vision—the mental model—is a vision that people become committed to because it reflects their personal views. It uplifts aspirations, gives courage, and fosters risk taking. The shared vision becomes the overarching goal (pp. 200-209).

Discipline Focus Within
an Interdisciplinary Environment

All health care disciplines are concerned with promoting health, well-being, and development. Thus, much of health care is provided within an interdisciplinary environment. However, each professional practitioner has a mental model of the service he or she is providing. Each discipline has a particular focus. This focus of concern is referred to as the *proper object*. Identifying the proper object of a practice field is one approach to begin describing the specialized knowledge of that field and thereby to identify and measure its contribution to society and evaluate the effectiveness of the services offered.

Object refers to that which is studied or observed, and *proper* is used in the sense of belonging to the field. Medicine is concerned with illness and health and the prevention and treatment of illnesses. Psychology is concerned with behavior and learning experiences, and particularly with variations in learning and behavior. Nursing is concerned with caring for persons when they are unable to care for themselves or lack the knowledge to do so.

When the proper object of each health-related professional service is known, the domains and boundaries of the professions can be described. Roles and responsibilities can then be allocated and tasks assigned appropriately. This kind of differentiation is important to the planning phase of service delivery and has practical implications for the design of operational components.

For example, because all health professions are concerned with the health of community members and the services required to achieve and maintain a healthy state, some of the data collected in a needs assessment are common to all of the professions. Common raw data include such items as age, sex, conditions of living, health state, education, socioeconomic information, cultural information, and family systems data. This is the basis for the movement toward developing a "common" record in health care agencies. However, the meaning attached to the data varies depending on the focus of concern of the discipline examining the data. There are also some discipline-specific data that provide information specific to the proper object of the discipline.

A look at how the data are used reveals that the use depends on the focus of concern or proper object of the discipline. The epidemiologist uses the data to determine morbidity and mortality patterns in various age groups. The focus of concern of the epidemiologist is the incidence of risk factors, incidence of illnesses, and causes of mortality in the community. The cardiologist's focus of concern is the incidence, identification, treatment, and prevention of cardiovascular diseases and with causative factors of morbidity and mortality related to the cardiovascular system. Although the two professionals may be using the same data, they are trying to answer different but related questions. The cardiologist is interested in the conclusions drawn by the epidemiologist but uses the data to answer different questions than the epidemiologist does. The cardiologist is interested primarily in treatment and efficacy of various treatments. The cardiologist recognizes the contribution of the epidemiologist and vice versa. However, the cardiologist does not try to be an epidemiologist. Though the incidence of cardiovascular disease and the efficacy of various treatment protocols are of interest to the nurse, the primary focus of nursing is the management of the self-care system of persons who have cardiovascular problems or the potential for developing them.

The emphasis in recent years on the interdisciplinary aspects of care is referred to frequently in this book. Caution is required that this emphasis does not shift to becoming a nondisciplinary emphasis. *Interdisciplinarity* means professionals working together in a cooperative, complementary fashion, each profession bringing a particular knowledge base and skill set to the situation. In a nondisciplinary environment, it is assumed that one professional can replace another. This approach does not recognize the focus of concern or proper object, the knowledge base, the skill set, and the experience peculiar to each profession. Organizations that take the time to specify the focus of concern or domain and boundaries of each of the health care professions have a frame of reference for determining roles and responsibilities and can specify the nature of the services required and the outcomes expected from provision of that service.

Nursing—the Invisible Service?

When and why is nursing required in a community? Nursing is often referred to as the "silent service." The absence of nursing is recognized, but the projected and even the actual need for nursing is more difficult to describe. Since the early 1900s with the movement of nursing out of the community and into the hospital, nursing has been inextricably linked to the practice of medicine, and it still is today in some settings. Nurses are often viewed as the handmaidens of physicians. It is taken for granted by health care enterprises that patients/clients will be provided with "nursing care," but the "essence" of nursing is not defined or clearly understood. In many settings, because nurses tend to be available 24 hours a day, 7 days a week, they frequently fill in for other workers, so that time is taken away from the essential nursing tasks. Although much of the care required by patients/clients of health care enterprises is nursing, decisions regarding admission, discharge, and transfer are frequently decisions made by physicians on the basis of medical criteria, and much of nursing activity requires a physician order. Reference in the nursing literature to the independent, dependent, and interdependent aspects of nursing practice reflects the struggle of the nursing profession to describe the domain of nursing for members of the profession and for the public at large.

Within the work world, nursing is the invisible entity. Over the past 15 years, because the nursing profession has had such difficulty describing what nursing is about, nursing has been systematically eliminated from positions of decision making and policy formulation under any number of "covers" (C. Estabrookes, personal communication, 1997). The director of nursing or vice president of nursing has frequently been replaced with a director or vice president of patient care, with no requirement that this person be a nurse, although the number of contact hours between nursing staff and patients/clients is greater than that between the patient/client and any other care provider. In these settings, the tasks of nursing can be identified, but the essence of the service cannot be described, so professional nurses are being replaced with nonprofessional workers who are able to perform the same "task" but are not able to provide "nursing." Havens (1998), in comparing the 1994 level of involvement of nursing in hospital governance to the 1990 level, found that nurses are not as involved in policy making as classic studies and organizational experts recommend. More nursing involvement is needed on both finance committees and governing bodies.

With the expansion of nursing education in the universities, the development of doctoral programs and programs of research, and certification of various nursing specialties requiring advanced nursing education, nursing may be emerging as an entity separate from that of assistant to the physician. Fagin (1996) noted that in some jurisdictions nursing now is being given the authority to admit and discharge patients to institutions and health care programs on the basis of the need for nursing. There is also a move to develop nursing centers. In some situations, the purpose of the center is provision of nursing (Michaels, 1991). In other instances, these centers are primarily substitutes for physician services. Ensuring that a place is truly a nursing center requires specifying the proper object of nursing, identifying the domain and boundaries, and describing the services rather than just identifying nursing tasks (Barrett, 1993).

In the health care enterprise, much of the work of professional practitioners and particularly nursing practice is under the direct control of the enterprise through the policies, procedures, documentation structures, and so on. Although the people designing and developing these structures may not realize it, the components are developed from the mental models of nursing held by the persons developing them. At the present stage of nursing as a professional practice discipline, despite the American Nurses Association's definition of nursing, there is no clear mental model commonly accepted in the United States, Canada, or elsewhere in the world for nursing. This does not negate the need for and utility of making explicit the mental model in operation within individual health care settings. A mental model of nursing practice exists for every nurse. It may not be explicitly defined. It may not be theoretically congruent. However, it does exist, and nurses practice from it. When nurses within a health care enterprise share a mental model and this model becomes expressed in the clinical information system, it can be shared with others for the improvement of patient services. Models representative of persons' engagement in health care are derived from the study of persons in such situations. Models representative of nursing practice can be derived from the study of nursing practice situations and the development of theories of nursing practice. Unfortunately, the education of many nurses did not include nursing theory, and consequently nurses do not recognize the contribution that such theories can make to the development of nursing practice and to nursing knowledge.

The need for nursing is directly related to the nature of persons' engagement in health care. Engagement in health care can take one of three forms:

1. Acting on one's own behalf in health-related matters—self-care
2. Assisting another or being a caregiver for another, whether one does this alone or with other caregivers
3. Caring for oneself or for another with the help of one or more health professionals

The focus in the remainder of this chapter is on developing models of self-care and care of dependent persons and relating them to nursing.

A Model of Self-Care

Definition of Self-Care

Self-care has been defined in many ways in the literature. In this book, the definition of self-care is consistent with that proposed by Orem (1995). The reader is referred to the writings of Orem for a more detailed discussion of the topics that follow. Self-care is activity performed by mature or maturing persons within a time frame to maintain life, to facilitate healthful functioning, and to promote continuing personal development and well-being. Self-care, as the term is being used in this book, is a function of being human, is action that is purposeful and deliberate, has a time orientation, and is health related.

Self-care activities are learned and take place within a particular sociocultural context. It is important that persons designing, implementing, or evaluating a health care service be aware of and incorporate the cultural values and beliefs of the target population. When health care providers do not consider culture, programs may not be accessed or may not be effective. For example, provision of prenatal services has long been recognized as an effective means of improving morbidity and mortality statistics for mothers and newborns. However, one health agency attempting to provide these services to an immigrant population found that attendance was not what was expected. On exploring why, the agency found that the culture of the women of the target population disapproved of women going out in public without a male member of the family; therefore, the women were prevented from attending the prenatal program. On the positive side, health agencies have found that taking the prenatal services to the streets via vans or blood pressure clinics to shopping malls is very successful.

The social context is also important. If health promotion programs such as those promoting smoking cessation or use of condoms to prevent the spread of sexually transmitted disease do not take into consideration the peer pressure and social environment of the target population, they will be much less effective than the proponents of the programs predicted.

Viewing the social and cultural context as a conditioning factor of self-care has implications for the strategies that health care workers choose to effect a change in self-care behaviors that are considered inappropriate. Educating people in new ways of looking after themselves must be done in a culturally and economically sensitive manner. In many instances, rather than providing education, it may be more appropriate to bring about economic or environmental changes, or even to address cultural beliefs on a community basis. Although the target is to ensure that the self-care behaviors are appropriate, the intervention or action required to bring this about may be on a community or family level rather than at the individual level (Edwards, Cere, & Leblond, 1993).

Self-care is a function of demand. Although there are certain general demands to be met—for example, to maintain a sufficient intake of food—the specifics of the demand vary with a number of factors, including age, gender, and health state. These are identified more specifically in Figure 2.1. Accomplishing self-care is a function of capability to do so, or self-care agency.

The Processes of Self-Care

The processes of self-care are embodied in three sets of operations: estimative, transitional, and productive operations. Each of these sets of operations has specific abilities associated with it.

The estimative operations are cognitive. They involve being aware that some action is required and acquiring information about the various courses of action that are appropriate. One must have some understanding of the goals to be achieved and of the means to achieve those goals. For example, as persons reach

30

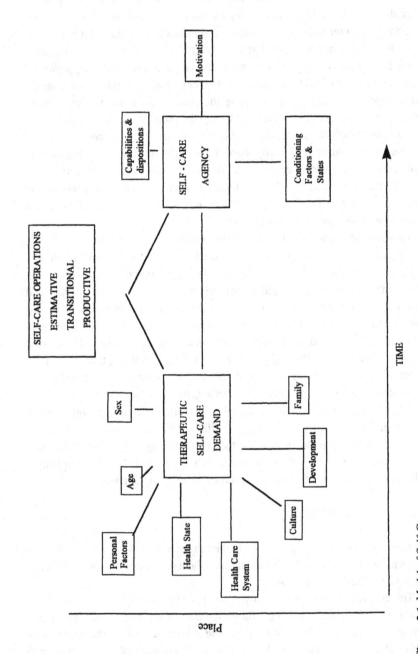

Figure 2.1. Model of Self-Care
SOURCE: Derived from Orem (1995).

adulthood, they usually understand the necessity to health of maintaining a balance between rest and activity and ways of achieving this—sleeping 8 hours a night, resting in a sitting position when short of breath, walking 2 miles each day, and so on. Evaluating the options available for achieving the desired goals is a part of this operation.

The transitional operations are also cognitive, involving reflecting on, comparing, and choosing between optional courses of action. These operations involve understanding cause and effect: "If I do this, such and such will be the result; if I do that, so and so will be the result." The choices that are available and that one chooses to make are influenced by conditioning factors such as value system, availability of resources, and environment.

The productive operations are both cognitive and psychomotor. They include securing resources, following a specified course of action, monitoring for results, and making judgments about continuing a course of action or returning to estimative operations. They also include some motivational and value-related components and physical capabilities to perform required actions.

Although these three sets of operations are related, a person can successfully complete one or more types of operation without being able to complete all three. For instance, a quadriplegic person can have an understanding of the self-care required and make choices about what is to be done but be unable to actually perform the required self-care. In other cases, a person may be able to do the self-care after another person makes the decision about the course of action to be followed.

Summary of the Model of Self-Care

In summary, as depicted in Figure 2.1, self-care is a function of the inter-relationships among conditioning factors, demands for self-care, and self-care capabilities. It consists of estimative, transitional, and productive operations that occur within a time-place frame of reference.

A Model of Caring for
Another—Dependent Care

Engagement in health care can also take the form of caring for another. Considering the current trends in health care services, this has significant implications for design of health care services. People are discharged earlier from acute care facilities, and skilled nursing care is expensive and is being replaced by family members. Identifying the care that people require and the skills that family members must have to provide that care is an important part of any health care delivery system. If the learning needs of family members are not addressed, the patient does not receive the care required and is readmitted to the services of the health care agency, often with preventable complications. The concept of dependent care, which is a part of self-care deficit nursing theory, is useful to nurses and to administrators in determining the requirements of dependent persons for assistance and the ability of the caregivers to meet those requirements. This information can be used to structure discharge and transfer processes, procedures, and documentation to facilitate a smooth transition from inpatient facility to the home and community (see Chapter 7 of this book).

Definition of Dependent Care

Dependent care is care that is performed on a continuing basis for a period of time on behalf of socially dependent persons, including children or disabled persons, that contributes to their health and well-being (Orem, 1995). Dependent care may be provided to a single individual by one person or by a number of persons. Although dependent care is usually thought of as being provided by an adult, M. J. Denyes (personal communication, 1997), in working with inner-city children, found that occasionally children would assume adult responsibilities and become the caregiver for less responsible parents.

Dependent care is also a form of deliberate action. The purpose to be achieved through dependent care is meeting the care requirements of a socially dependent person who is unable to accomplish his or her own self-care. The operations related to dependent care are the same as those related to self-care: knowing, decision making, and production of care. However, the capabilities and motivation required to carry out these operations are different in that the actions are directed at another and the requirements for care arise from the frame of reference of the dependent person.

The Processes of Dependent Care

Parallel to self-care, dependent care involves three sets of operations: estimative, transitional, and productive. However, in dependent care, the dependent and the caregiver(s) carry out the operations together. The extent of involvement of the dependent varies with the development and operability of that person's self-care agency.

Estimative operations have both cognitive and interpersonal components. In cooperation with the dependent, the caregiver needs to be able to determine the care that is required (the therapeutic self-care demand of the dependent) and to modify the prescription of actions to be taken to meet that demand on an ongoing basis. This requires having an understanding of the array of appropriate actions available to be taken to meet the self-care demand and also being able and willing to communicate with the dependent to determine which is the best course of action from the perspective of the dependent. The ability to understand a situation from the perspective of another is important.

The transitional operations involve decision making and are also cognitive and interpersonal, including working with the dependent to arrive at a mutual decision about a desired course of action. This is true even when the reaction of the dependent is nonverbal, as in the case of small infants. Through crying and avoidance behaviors, they can communicate their likes and dislikes to caregivers. As an action system evolves, the dependent may wish to change the system, and the caregiver then needs to know how to manage the desire for change. Again, communication and perceiving the situation from the perspective of the dependent are important, along with the capability of the caregiver to be responsive and flexible.

The production operations are both psychomotor and interpersonal. Production of dependent care involves perhaps the greatest variation in skills from those associated with self-care. The actions and associated capabilities required include some or all of the following: the interpersonal skills to facilitate and to complement the activities that the dependent person engages in to care for him- or herself, working with the body of another, assembling and managing resources, coordinating actions among a group of caretakers, and integrating care of another into the daily care of self.

Summary of Dependent Care

In summary, as depicted in Figure 2.2, dependent care is a function of the interrelationships among the self-care deficit of the dependent, the capability of the caregiver (dependent care agency), the self-care demand, and conditioning factors of the caregiver(s). It also consists of estimative, transitional, and productive operations that occur within a time-place frame of reference.

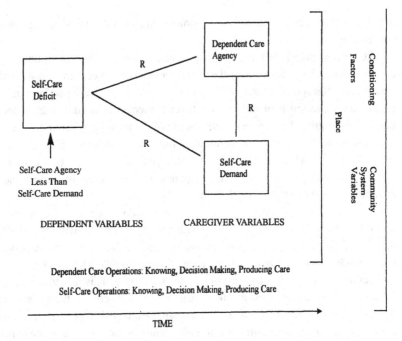

Figure 2.2. Model of Dependent Care
SOURCE: Derived frrom Orem (1995).

Multiple Caregivers in a Dependent Care System

When more than one caregiver is involved, the care system becomes more complicated. The dependent is required to interact with a number of caregivers. The nature of the care system changes with the variations in interpersonal dynamics as the caregiver changes and the dependent person is required to accommodate the variations in the personal characteristics of the caregivers, communication skills, conditioning factors, and capability as a caregiver. There may be a need for specifying a course of action that all caregivers will follow. Being able to assess the capabilities of each caregiver and to develop a course of action that maximizes the effectiveness of each when multiple persons are involved is an additional required capability.

In addition to being a caregiver for another, the dependent care agent is engaged in self-care. The literature on caregiver burden and burnout makes reference to the problems caregivers have in maintaining their own health and

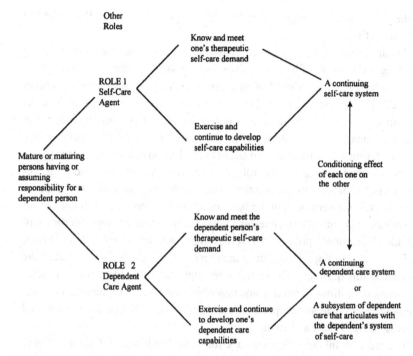

Figure 2.3. Roles of Dependent Care Agents

SOURCE: From *Nursing: Concepts of Practice* (5th ed.), by D. E. Orem, 1995, St. Louis, MO: Mosby Year-Book. Copyright 1995 by Mosby Year-Book. Reprinted with permission.

energy and dealing with their own needs while attending to the dependent person. The dual roles of the dependent care agent are illustrated in Figure 2.3.

The Domain of Nursing

The Proper Object of Nursing

Self-care and dependent care can exist without assistance from health professionals. When professionals become involved, their activities articulate with self-care and/or dependent care, forming a new action system. As described earlier, each profession has a particular focus of concern that is the basis of its relationship with the person requiring care or with the caregivers. The actions of the professionals, caregivers, and persons requiring care are all interrelated and interactive.

An important question implied in the health care literature and plaguing planning and delivery of health services over the years has been, "Is this patient or this subpopulation in need of nursing, or will some other type of worker suffice?" The profession has tried to answer this question by describing the tasks that nurses can and cannot do and by describing features of nursing practice in such statements as the American Nurses Association's (1994) social policy statement. Employers have tried to answer the question through job descriptions and policy statements specifying roles and activities. Society has tried to answer this question through nurse practice acts, which again describe the tasks of nursing. Nursing service settings have developed statements of beliefs about nursing and associated objectives as a frame of reference for services they will provide. Educational programs have developed similar statements to provide direction for selecting of content in the nursing curricula. Nurse theorists have also asked this question. Their efforts are reported in the literature in articles proposing definitions of nursing and describing the essence of nursing as caring (Leininger, 1984), as an interpersonal process (Peplau, 1992), as an interactional process (King, 1992), and so on.

The most useful definition we have found to date is that of Dorothea Orem (1995). Observing nurses in practice, she asked herself, "What condition exists in a person when judgements are made that persons should be under nursing care?" (p. 8). She came to the conclusion that the condition is "the inability of persons to provide continuously for themselves that amount and quality of required self-care because of situations of personal health" (p. 8), or, in the case of children, the inability of parents or guardians to provide the required self-care. This she refers to as the proper object of nursing. This definition has proven useful in providing a basis for continuing development in which the patient variables of concern to nursing have been identified, operational definitions have been developed, research programs have begun, information systems have been developed, outcomes of nursing services have been identified, and quality assurance programs have been designed, as illustrated throughout this book.

The Articulation of Self-Care and Dependent Care With Nursing

Models of individuals' engagement in health care and care of dependent others have been described. In this section, we will look at how the engagement of persons in health-related care articulates with the service called nursing.

Consistent with self-care deficit nursing theory, nursing is concerned with health-related self-care/dependent care systems; how well they are accomplishing the goal of promotion of health, well-being, and development; what changes need to be put in place; and what capabilities need to be developed to accomplish the goals (Orem, 1995). Orem proposed that the product of nursing is the development of a nursing system, which is an action system composed of the actions and interactions of nurse(s) and patient(s) or client(s), the purpose of which is meeting the therapeutic self-care demand of the patient(s) or client(s) within a specified time-place frame of reference and providing for meeting this demand in the future.

The Variables of Concern to Nursing

The variables of concern to nursing in accomplishing the purposes of nursing are identified in the models of self-care and dependent care. The role of nursing in relation to the design and implementation of systems of self-care/dependent care includes

- Identifying the conditioning factors that are actively affecting or conditioning the current situation or that may become potentially active
- Relating conditioning factors to general requirements for self-care to determine the appropriate action system in the specific situation (calculating the therapeutic self-care demand)
- Participating in the design of self-care systems for individuals and for populations
- Evaluating self-care capability in relation to demand
- Evaluating dependent-care capability required in the situation
- Facilitating the development of self-care/dependent care capabilities
- Managing the exercise of self-care capabilities of the patient/client and facilitating/participating in meeting the therapeutic self-care demand of the patient/client

Note that the role of nursing has been stated in relation to self-care or dependent care systems. It has not been described, for example, in terms of management of pathological states, administering medications, performing procedures, or teaching the patient/caregiver, although these may be activities in which the nurse engages. This is a significant variation in framing the interaction between nurses and patient/clients. Describing nursing's role in this way provides administrators with a different mental model of nursing and with a different perspective for evaluating the cost-effectiveness of nursing programs.

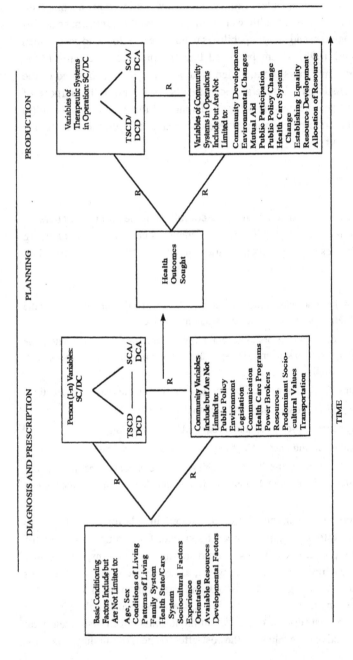

Figure 2.4. Variables of Concern to Nursing

SOURCE: From "Orem's General Theory of Nursing and Community Nursing," by S. G. Taylor and K. McLaughlin, 1991, *Nursing Science Quarterly*, 4(4), pp. 153-160. Adapted with permission.

NOTE: SC, self-care; DC, dependent care; TSCD, therapeutic self-care demand; DCD, dependent care demand; SCA, self-care agency; DCA, dependent care agency.

38

TABLE 2.1   Selected Components of Therapeutic Self-Care Demand (TSCD) and Role Responsibilities

TSCD Component of Self-Care System	Physician	Nurse	Social Worker	Other
Maintain a sufficient intake of air	Prescribe medication, oxygen therapy	Administer meds, oxygen, teach therapies Monitor pulmonary status	Resources for home oxygen administration	Resp.therapist— set up equipment, monitor, administer oxygen, medications
Maintain a sufficient intake of food, water	Prescribe	Administer feed, position Monitor intake Teach		Dietician— consult
Provide care re: elimination	Order, e.g., catheters, medications	Administer, monitor, provide skin care, other care		
Maintain balance between rest and activity	Prescribe medications	Establish schedule, administer medications Implement pain/rest strategies Implement activity plan Evaluate knowledge of strategies and teach Identify appropriate activities		OT or recreational therapist— establish activity program, physio program
Maintain a balance between solitude and social interaction		Establish schedule, implement plan Evaluate knowledge of strategies and teach	Resources for social interaction	Recreational therapist— participate with nursing in establishing plan, implementing
Prevent hazards		Identify risk factors Develop and implement appropriate plan		
Promote normalcy		Identify nterferences, Develop plan Implement plan	Family counseling	

It also gives direction for the kind of patient data that must be collected to determine if the purposes of nursing are being achieved and provides direction for developing guidelines related to evaluating the performance of individual nurses as well as the performance of nursing service as a whole.

The variables of concern to nursing and processes associated with production of nursing are illustrated in Figure 2.4.

The Complementary Relationship of Nursing to the Activities of Other Health Care Professionals

Much of nursing is carried out in cooperation with other health care professionals. To illustrate the complementary relationship of health care professionals within an interdisciplinary environment, Table 2.1 compares the role of the nurse with that of some health care personnel in reference to selected elements of the therapeutic self-care demand at a particular point in time. Developing an understanding of the proper object (focus of concern) of the disciplines involved and expanding on the concerns of nursing through development of a mental model of nursing make it possible to differentiate the role of nursing and the articulation between nursing and other professions in the health care setting.

Summary

In this chapter, the importance of mental models to the health care enterprise is addressed. Models for individuals' engagement in health care and the articulation of these models with nursing are presented. The models show the "what" of nursing—what nursing is all about. The result of this articulation is an understanding of when and why nursing is required. Use of these models in the design and delivery of nursing services will be elaborated on in subsequent chapters.

References

American Nurses Association. (1994). *Nursing's social policy statement*. Kansas City, MO: Author.

Barrett, E. A. (1993). Nursing centres without nursing frameworks: What's wrong with this picture. *Nursing Science Quarterly, 6*(3), 115-117.

Edwards, N., Cere, M., & Leblond, D. (1993). A community based intervention to prevent falls among seniors. *Family and Community Health, 15*(4), 57-65.

Fagin, C. M. (1996). Executive leadership: Improving nursing practice, education, and research. *Journal of Nursing Administration, 26*(3), 30-37.

Havens, D. S. (1998). An update on nursing involvement in hospital governance 1990-1996. *Nursing Economics$, 18,* 6-11.

King, I. M. (1992). King's theory of goal attainment. *Nursing Science Quarterly, 5,* 19-26.

Leininger, M. (1984). Caring: A central focus of nursing and health services. In M. Leininger (Ed.), *Care: The essence of nursing and health.* Thorofare, NJ: Slack.

Michaels, C. M. (1991). A nursing HMO: 10 months with Carondelet St. Mary's Hospital-based nurse case management. *Aspen's Advisor for Nurse Executives, 6,*(11), 1-4.

Orem, D. E. (1995). *Nursing: Concepts of practice* (5th ed.). St. Louis, MO: Mosby Year-Book.

Peplau, H.E. (1992). Interpersonal relations: A theoretical framework for application in nursing practice. *Nursing Science Quarterly, 5,* 13-18.

Senge, P. M. (1990). *The fifth discipline: The art and practice of the learning organization.* New York: Doubleday.

Taylor, S. G., & McLaughlin, K. (1991). Orem's general theory of nursing and community nursing. *Nursing Science Quarterly, 4,* 153-160.

CHAPTER 3

Models for Nursing Administration

Within a health care enterprise, there may be a body of nurses designated as "nursing administration," or this function may be dispersed throughout the organization and assigned to a number of persons, both nursing and non-nursing. In either situation, if an enterprise offers health care services to the public, there must be an overall understanding of the service being offered, and certain functions of administration relative to that service must be carried out. As described in Chapter 2, it is the thesis of this book that provision of nursing services in the 21st century requires that persons charged with ensuring the delivery of the service have a theoretical and practical understanding of nursing as well as an understanding of theory and practice associated with administration. In this chapter, an overview of the nature of organizations is presented. This is followed by a model depicting the dimensions of nursing as an entity within the overall health care enterprise. Nursing administration is then defined, and administrative structures and functions of organizations specific to nursing are described. An integration of the variables significant to the practice of nursing as specified in self-care deficit nursing theory and those significant to administration within a health care enterprise is proposed as a model for nursing administration. The need for a mental model of nursing within the health care enterprise becomes clear when examined against a background of understandings about organizations.

Nature of Organizations

Definition of Organization

An organization is a cooperative system in itself and a subset of a larger cooperative system called society. Barnard (1962) has defined an organization as "a system of consciously coordinated activities or forces of two or more persons" (p. 73). In other words, an organization is made up of the activities of human beings. "An organization comes into being when (1) there are persons able to communicate with each other (2) who are willing to contribute action (3) to accomplish a common purpose" (Barnard, 1962, p. 81). Barnard concluded that the elements of an organization therefore are communication, willingness to serve, and common purpose.

Without a willingness of persons to act cooperatively, there can be no organization. In other words, persons must be willing to give up some measure of personal control to work together. This willingness to cooperate may fluctuate at various times. It involves balancing sacrifices with satisfactions. The satisfactions may come from inducements offered by the enterprise, such as monetary compensation or personal recognition, or they may be the fulfillment of some personal goal. These individual motives and what satisfies them are subject to influences that originate outside the particular health care enterprise, for each person is a member of more than one organization or cooperative system at any one time and is being influenced by all systems in which he or she is participating.

Organizations commonly develop a mission statement or goal(s) to share with all persons associated with the enterprise as a means of clarifying the purpose of the enterprise. Working toward a common purpose is much less complicated in a simple organization or when an enterprise exists for a single purpose such as providing shelter for the homeless. In a complex organization such as a health care enterprise, although an overall common purpose may be stated, the common purposes of the subunits within the organization must be consistent with that overall common purpose. For example, although the primary purpose of the health care enterprise is delivery of health care services to patients/clients, there is variation among the health care professionals providing that service, between the health care professionals and administration, and between the recipients of the service and the providers about what constitutes achievement of that purpose and how that purpose is to be achieved. These enterprises also are in the "business" of education in that they provide clinical experiences for all of the health care professions and for the professions concerned with health care administration, in some cases developing and delivering the educational program. They are in the "business" of research and knowledge development in that they are the gateway to and a repository of a clinical database essential to the development of new treatment and care strategies and essential to the development of the knowledge base of health care professions, particularly the nursing profession. Some of these enterprises are also in the "business" of providing residential services and assistance in daily living. Each "business" is represented in the enterprise by a different cooperative system, each one interacting with every other one.

To further complicate matters, some of the persons providing services are employees of the enterprise, and others are given privileges to practice their profession within the domain of the enterprise. Assessment of what should be the cost of conducting the business and the amount of funds available for the capital and operating expenses of the enterprise is frequently wholly or certainly partially determined by outside entities such as governments and insurance providers, whose primary "business" is governing or maintaining a profitable insurance company, not delivering health care. Even the services that an enterprise is allowed to provide or must provide may be determined by such systems outside the enterprise.

Furthermore, within each cooperative system or organizational unit, although persons may espouse a common purpose, each of these persons has an individual perspective in relation to that purpose. This individual understanding is based on the sum total of the person's current and previous experiences. The operational understanding of the purpose or mission statement of the enterprise and of the subgroups to which each person belongs varies. In addition, each person is a part of other organizations—professional, religious, personal—that also influence his or her understanding of and willingness to act in relation to the common purpose. Presentations made by nurse administrators at nursing theory/nursing practice conferences indicate that when the common purpose includes a shared mental model of nursing, the associated allocation of resources to foster this shared understanding and common purpose strengthens organizational effectiveness and enhances staff loyalty and job satisfaction.

To achieve a cooperative effort, a purpose must be shared throughout the organization. Without communication, it is impossible to achieve cooperative action. Communication includes the use of language as well as nonverbal techniques. Understanding intention as well as words is significant in achieving cooperative action.

Communication of the common purpose is reflected in the mission statement, the employment policies, the programs that are developed, the recording system related to service delivery, the staff orientation and education programs, and the marketing and public relations program of the enterprise. Organizational structure is also a major consideration in the communication process. The structure can facilitate or interfere with communication.

Factors That Influence Organizational Structure

■ Physical Environment

The physical environment influences the nature of the organizational structure in a number of ways. Keeping in mind that the purpose of the structure is to promote achievement of common purpose, willingness to serve, and communication, the most appropriate structure will be different if the services are centered in one location, are provided from a number of regional locations, or are totally decentralized, as in provision of home care services.

The physical environment may serve as an inducement to work or may provide a focus of dissatisfaction. There is much emphasis today on the ergonomics of the workplace. This emphasis in the public press influences employee attitudes and acceptance regarding perceived acceptable or unacceptable physical settings. If the physical environment cannot be changed and is a source of dissatisfaction, restructuring the organization to give the employee greater satisfaction in another aspect (such as more input into policy making) may be required.

■ Social Environment

Recognizing the need for social compatibility and accommodating that need should be considered in determining organizational structure. Social incompatibility can be a major deterrent to cooperative effort. The incompatibilities may be associated with culture, language, education, personal ambition, religion, social status, and so on. Barnard (1962) suggested that when there is lack of compatibility, both formal and informal communication become difficult in the organization and may even be impossible.

■ *Individuals*

Because a cooperative system is made up of the actions of persons, it becomes self-evident that employing, unemploying, and situating the right person in the right place at the right time to carry out the business of an enterprise are key to successfully accomplishing the purpose of the enterprise. The availability of the "right" person or persons influences the structure of the organization, as does the nature or characteristics of the persons who are available.

■ *Specialization of the Organization*

There are essentially five bases for specialization of organizations (Barnard, 1962). These are identified below with specific reference to the health care enterprise.

1. The place where work is done—for example, acute care, community, emergency room, outpatient clinic
2. The time at which the work is done—day shift, night shift, 24-hour coverage
3. The persons with whom work is done—nurses, physicians, environmental officers
4. The objects on which work is done—children, adults
5. The method or process by which work is done—surgery, medical therapy, nursing care

■ *The Functions to Be Performed*

Form should follow function. The functions of human service organizations originate in the needs of the population served and include governance of the entity, administration of the operation, and the essential operational functions, including distribution, production, and financing of services. Performance of each of these functions requires provision of equipment and supplies, facilities, and personnel. The content of the essential operations varies with the nature of the service to be provided. The interrelationship of these functions is illustrated in Figure 3.1.

■ *The Complexity of the Organization*

The more complex the organization, the greater the number of organizational units that can coexist. There are any number of possibilities for arranging these

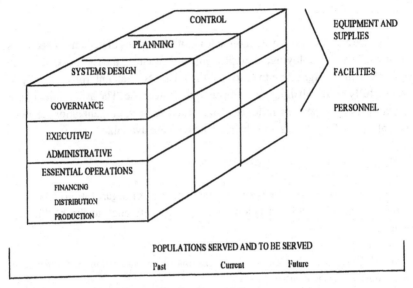

Figure 3.1. Functions of Human Service Organizations

organizational units while still accomplishing the purpose of the organization. Conceptualizing the health care enterprise as an organization composed of multiple organizational units is helpful in understanding its complexity and the operations necessary to achieve its purpose and in considering the possible variations in structure of personnel that can facilitate accomplishing the purposes of the enterprise. The challenges today are to design cost-effective organizational structures that are "seamless" from the perspective of the patient/client and to facilitate accomplishing the functions of administration, including coordination of the activities of patients/clients, professional personnel, and support personnel. This requires an organization that is vertically, horizontally, and functionally integrated (Shortell, Gillies, Anderson, Erickson, & Mitchell, 1996). Issues of coordination versus integration must be addressed if progress is to be made in accomplishing clinical integration across the continuum of care and functional integration, including strategic planning, information systems, quality control, financial control, and management of human resources. Although there has been a great deal of structural reorganization of health care enterprises, little research has been done in the health care industry to determine the advantages and disadvantages of the various structures that have been implemented. It is timely to consider the role of nursing theory in facilitating this integration while maintaining the integrity of the nursing services.

Nursing Administration

Nursing Administration Defined

Nursing administration as defined by Orem (1995) is

the body of persons who function in situational contexts to collectively manage courses of affairs enabling for the provision of nursing for the population currently being served by an organized health service institution or agency and for populations to be served at future times. (p. 395)

Whereas individual practitioners of nursing primarily are concerned with providing nursing to individuals or groups of individuals (i.e., a caseload), nursing administration is concerned with designing, planning, and producing nursing for populations and subpopulations of persons requiring nursing. Orem (1989) identified the difference between the two in terms of their "proper object," the particular focus of each. The individual nursing practitioner's object of concern is "persons who seek and can benefit from nursing because of the presence of existent or predicted health derived or health related self-care or dependent care deficits" (p. 56; see Chapter 2 of this book). The proper object of nursing administration is "the definable but changing population of persons for whom a legally constituted enterprise ensures the continuing availability and actual provision of nursing" (p. 56).

Dimensions of the Entity "Nursing"
Within the Larger System

Persons responsible for the design and delivery of nursing services must be able to conceptualize the whole organizational schema of a health care enterprise and the place of nursing within it. In other words, they must see the "big picture" of nursing as an organizational entity within a larger organizational system, as laid out in Figure 3.2. This figure is an adaptation of a model developed by Dorothea Orem for a nursing practice project at The Johns Hopkins Hospital

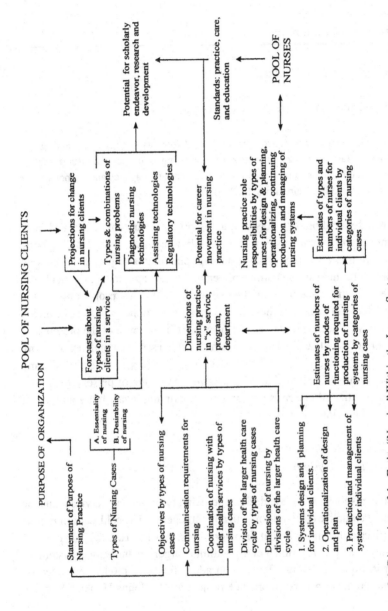

Figure 3.2. Dimensions of the Entity "Nursing" Within the Larger System
SOURCE: Allison (1977).

(Allison, 1977, pp. 50-51). The dimensions and their relationships depicted in this model can serve as the basis for strategic planning for nursing within an organization, as demonstrated in subsequent chapters.

The model directs attention to

1. The purposes of the organization
2. The purposes of nursing
3. The types of nursing cases (populations to be served)
4. Forecasting and projecting the types of nursing problems in relation to the nursing technologies needed
5. Types and numbers of nurses needed to manage nursing problems forecasted
6. Communication systems
7. Coordination of services
8. Design of nursing systems
9. Production of nursing through operationalization of designs
10. Career pathways
11. Research and development

In examining the model, it becomes clear that each of the components is interrelated and that if changes occur in one component, other parts and the whole may be affected as well. The substance or content of each of these components is derived from the mental model of nursing that is held by both nurses and non-nurses who are responsible for and contribute to the design, implementation, and evaluation of the nursing service. Without a clearly defined mental model for nursing that is understood and shared by persons responsible for the service, each of the above components will be developed in isolation, making it difficult to monitor the overall nursing program for efficiency and effectiveness. Figure 3.3 further elaborates on the conceptualization of the health care enterprise as a collection of organizational units of which nursing could be a part.

In this book, we are proposing that a mental model for nursing provides the common purpose that unites nursing as an entity across a number of organizational units. This is necessary to achieving clinical integration. The mental model provides the "glue" that holds together all of the components of the nursing service identified in Figure 3.3. The mental model or theory of nursing practice gives direction for identifying the nursing content relative to the functions of administration of the nursing services.

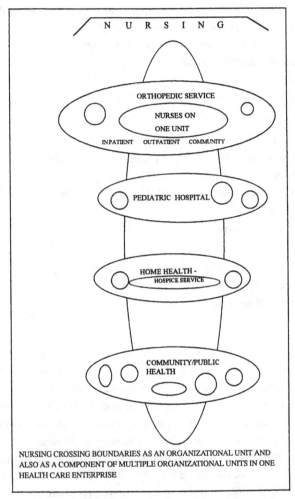

Figure 3.3. Variations in the Place of Nursing in the Organization

Nursing Administration and
the Operational Functions of the Organization

Administration of nursing within an organization includes contributing from a nursing perspective to the governing, administration, and operational functions of the organization. Responsibilities include

- Providing leadership in development of the mission and vision for the enterprise
- Informing the governing board about nursing's contribution to the enterprise
- Determining the needs for nursing based on the characteristics of the population being served
- Designing and planning for nursing operations, including the structuring and development of the practice of nursing within the organization in order to

    Design appropriate nursing systems to complement and facilitate implementation of self-care systems and dependent care systems

    Specify the contributory systems required (the equipment and supplies, facilities and physical plant, and personnel) to produce the nursing systems

    Inform the governing board of resources required

    Manage resources to ensure the distribution and availability of nursing services to the user

    Facilitate growth and development of nursing staff

- Facilitating research and development activities in relation to development of patient care technologies

Nursing administration must be able to articulate and communicate the nursing perspective, how nursing can and does contribute to the purposes of the organization, and how nursing relates to other components in the organization. This requires an ability to clearly describe and explain nursing as a form of care required by and provided for individuals in the populations to be served. What kind of nursing knowledge is required to provide the nursing needed, and what are the capabilities of the nurses for designing and producing the required care? What types and numbers of nursing personnel are needed to provide the nursing required? To clearly articulate, communicate, and meet requirements for nursing, nursing administration must know the nursing variables to be addressed, the self-care abilities and limitations of the patients/clients, the therapeutic self-care demands to be met, the types and extent of self-care deficits (see Chapter 2 of this book), the capabilities and limitations of the nurses, and the types and numbers of nurses required to provide the nursing needed. This requires extensive use of available information from both inside and outside the health care enterprise in the community at large. Analysis of available patient data, use of clinical databases, reports both formal and informal, observations from personal experiences and reports of others, and general information about health care and the community are all sources of information that must be used. All serve to enable nursing administration to determine and meet requirements for nursing and to present, discuss, dialogue, and plan with others strategies to meet the health care needs of the populations served. Program planning can best proceed with a mental vision, systems thinking, and a sound basis of information about the population to be served and the resources available and needed to provide the required care.

Articulation of a clearly defined mental model of nursing grounded in current nursing practice theory is the first step for nursing administration in providing leadership in the development of the mission and vision statement and laying the foundation for estimating nursing's contribution to the enterprise. In Chapter 2 of this book, such a mental model for nursing is described. The governing board cannot be expected to have a sufficient understanding of the services that various professionals are providing without input from those professionals. Without development of a vision and goals for nursing, there is no logical basis for understanding the contribution of nurses or for program development in relation to nursing services. This provides the foundation for the development of other structures such as the nursing component of the clinical information system, which in turn provides an essential database for program evaluation and for determining costs of the services provided.

In the past, nursing emphasized meeting all of a patient's needs, if possible, by providing "comprehensive" or "total" care. Due to changes in the health care system and the advent of managed care, health care services are driven less by management by objectives than by control of costs through resource utilization (Barnum & Kerfoot, 1995). The concern now is to prioritize services—to provide only those that are essential. Through definition of the focus of concern or proper object of nursing and the associated variables of concern to nursing and their interrelationships, nursing theory provides nursing administration with this direction. Without a nursing theory to provide such direction, nursing makes decisions based on management criteria or medical criteria. Neither is adequate for nursing.

Knowledge and skill in management and use of organization theory *provide no nursing basis* on which to structure and develop the practice of nursing to improve its product/service. Without a clear concept of what nursing produces and the outcomes or results to be expected from its services, can the nurse administrator truly develop and direct nursing practice? A strictly management focus may result in maintaining the status quo or making modifications by simply shifting things around—changing methods of delivery, for example. Many of these modifications, in the long run, may not be in the best interests of patients, nursing, and the organization. Knowing the focus and boundaries of nursing helps the nurse administrator to clarify and articulate the role, functions, and relationships of nursing to other health care services, thus facilitating and enhancing the contribution of each to the other and of all to the enterprise as a whole.

Source of Authority and Responsibility
for Nursing Administration

No matter what the organizational structure of the health care enterprise may be, authority and responsibility for nursing administration derives from two sources—delegated authority and the authority of knowledge. In the former, through the power granted by the governing body of the institution or agency for nursing, the nurse administrator acts to accomplish in whole or in part the purposes of the institution.

The authority of knowledge derives from knowing about nursing as a practice discipline and science, modes of delivery for production of nursing, and management—the design, production, and evaluation of nursing in relation to and in terms of its contribution to the whole of the enterprise. All is essential to delivery of quality nursing. For nurse administrators, authoritative knowledge derives from many sources. It includes but is not limited to educational preparation for nursing and administration, professional experience in practice and administration, leadership and managerial skills, and knowledge and understanding of organizations and organizational theory, the health care industry, and trends in the field. Authority of knowledge also derives from keeping informed—being current on developments in nursing knowledge and trends in the profession, the community, and the health care field in general. Such knowledge and continued learning for improvement and flexibility to meet the changes required for the 21st century are essential if nursing is to meet the needs of the future.

■ *The Knowledge Base for*
Administration of Nursing Services

The knowledge required by a person administrating nursing services can be likened to that of a production manager in the automobile manufacturing industry. That production manager must know what is being produced, what the automobile should look like, what it should be able to do, what processes are involved in production, how the time of workers should be managed to produce the product within budget allocations, what resources are required, and how to obtain and maintain a constant supply of those resources. Without that knowledge, the manager cannot do the job. To quote Orem (1989),

> Nursing administration is nursing oriented. This occurs through the nursing administrators' "dynamic knowing of nursing" and through their ability to think

nursing. Nursing administrators' judgements and decisions cannot be practical and rational unless these persons know nursing as a discipline of knowledge and practice both in relationship to their own work and to the work of nursing practitioners. (p. 62)

Many nurse administrators have an advanced understanding of management but lack both a clear conceptualization of why persons need nursing and an understanding of an organization's need for various advanced nursing practitioners to participate in the processes of design and delivery of nursing for patient populations. Haynor (1996) suggested that contemporary graduate education in nursing administration requires in-depth study of clinical nursing in addition to interdisciplinary and management courses.

The theme of this book is that an effective administrator of nursing services in the health world today must have an understanding of

1. The domain and boundaries of nursing as a discipline among other health care disciplines and the domains and boundaries of disciplines articulating with nursing
2. A practice philosophy to guide goal setting and evaluation
3. The process of identifying populations of concern to nursing
4. Designing nursing for individuals and for populations
5. The outcomes of nursing
6. Strategies for determining patient/client satisfaction

Nurse administrators also require a knowledge base related to the functions of administration, including

1. Communication and information management
2. Management of interpersonal relationships in an organization, including negotiations
3. Managing personnel for efficient service production
4. Financial management, including economics of the health care industry
5. Program development, implementation, and evaluation
6. Strategic management

■ *Integrating Practice and Management Goals*

Integrating the goals of professional practice and nursing management requires an understanding of nursing as a discipline of knowledge and a science, as well as an understanding of organization theory and economics, for all of these are foundational to nursing administration practice. Nyberg (1990) has identified a potential theoretic dichotomy between a physical/scientific, mechanistic, bureaucratic approach to administration and a more humanistic, perceptual, experiential approach. Given Barnard's (1962) concept of organization and the more modern view of Senge (1990) in terms of "the learning organization," these two perspectives can be brought together in nursing administration practice. A practice theory, such as the self-care deficit nursing theory, then, is both objective in the delineation of the nursing variables to be addressed and humanistic in value orientation. It can serve both quantitatively and qualitatively to integrate nursing practice and management goals.

If nursing is understood primarily in terms of organizing tasks and supervising people in performing them, then management of nursing practice will focus more on organizing service operations to get the tasks done. When the administrative focus is on nursing outcomes, clarifying the contribution of nursing to health care, and on leading, facilitating, and supporting nurses to improve nursing practice, both the objective and the humanistic perspectives are manifested.

From the self-care deficit nursing theory perspective, nursing goals are to overcome the identified actual or potential self-care deficits of the patient population being or to be served, the self-care limitations, and the factors negatively influencing both. Hence, with nursing goals clear, nursing management goals seek to organize, conduct, or produce nursing in light of them and to evaluate the processes and products—outcomes—of the production of nursing. This is done in terms of effectiveness, goals accomplished or not, and efficiency—goals achieved at least cost in terms of time, money, personnel, and so on. "Knowing nursing" provides direction for nursing management. It helps administrators of nursing services to describe and explain nursing in order to obtain results and thereby to obtain needed resources and to justify their utilization.

Model of Nursing Administration

The preceding discussion has made evident that the administration of nursing services requires the articulation of nursing theory and knowledge with administrative theory and knowledge. As illustrated throughout this book, a theory of nursing practice provides direction for understanding what the service called nursing is, for describing a population for nursing purposes, and for identifying the content relative to the administrative functions of the clinical service. Administration theory provides direction for specifying the functions of administration. Delivering quality nursing services to populations in an efficient, cost-effective manner requires understanding of both components.

Although the current trend in health care enterprises is to emphasize interdisciplinary activity, there still exists a service called nursing that is needed in society. Within a health care enterprise, there exists a cooperative system made up of nurses whose common purpose is provision of nursing to a particular population. As described previously, administration of this service may be vested in persons in a department or division of nursing or vested in a number of persons throughout the enterprise. The current trend in many enterprises to eliminate nurse administrator positions does not negate the need for fulfilling the functions associated with administration of the service, including developing the mental model of nursing to be provided by the organization, communicating the vision, structuring nursing practice to accomplish the goals of the organization, specifying the patient variables of concern to nursing within the information system, planning programs, ascertaining that the nursing contribution is evident, and justifying the need for nursing resources.

As the organization is "flattened" and emphasis is placed on interdisciplinary activity, the functions of nursing administration are distributed throughout the system and vested in many persons, some of whom may be nurses and others not. For example, in the cardiac surgical team, a physician may be the team leader and as such is responsible for ensuring that the administration functions related to nursing for the patients served by the cardiac team are performed.

It is important for all persons associated with the administration of the nursing service to understand what that service is and what outcomes can be expected as a result of provision of that service. Being able to state outcomes is one way of describing the service. Nursing tasks can be performed by many levels and categories of personnel. However, description from a nursing perspective of the population to be served, identification of the tasks to be performed, and design of a systematic plan of operations are the responsibilities of a professional nurse who cooperates with other health care professionals whose activities influence and are related to nursing.

In Table 3.1, a model is proposed that integrates nursing-specific components, derived in part from Orem's theory of nursing administration and the self-care deficit nursing theory, with the processes of administration. This model of nursing administration is applicable in a discipline-specific service delivery setting and in an interdisciplinary service delivery system. Subsequent chapters elaborate on the major components of this model. Descriptions of patient

TABLE 3.1   A Model of Administration Modified by Self-Care Deficit
Nursing Theory

Nursing	*Administration*
Nursing for Populations	
Continuous description of population for nursing purposes in terms of self-care deficits, self-care agency, basic conditioning factors, technologies	Selecting personnel (designers of self-care systems, caregivers, developers of practice technologies)
Calculation of what is required to provide nursing to populations; includes judgments about components of the therapeutic self-care demand, self-care agency, and the regulation of basic conditioning factors that may be required	Securing resources to support self-care (e.g., communication system, finances, materials, supplies, and facilities)
Production	Regulating production, evaluating production processes and outcomes
Nursing for Individuals	
Continuous description of changing needs and outcomes in terms of self-care deficits, self-care agency, basic conditioning factors	Leading/facilitating to achieve goals of self-care, including coordination of services and caregivers
Calculation of what is required to provide nursing to individuals	Structuring to achieve goals of self-care
Production	Regulating production, evaluating processes and outcomes

populations, utilization of nursing personnel, and structures and processes for implementing theory-based nursing are discussed along with practical applications.

Summary

The purpose of this chapter has been to describe the relationship between knowledge of nursing theory and the theory and knowledge associated with administration to facilitate delivery of the nursing component of health services. A conceptualization of the health care enterprise as a collection of cooperative systems of interaction or organization units coming together for a common purpose has been proposed. Nursing is a component of many of those organizational units. The utility of a theory of nursing practice to facilitate conceptualization of nursing as an entity throughout the health care enterprise has been discussed. Two models pertinent to nursing administration have been presented. One addresses the overall dimensions of nursing in an organization. The other focuses on the specific nursing variables of concern to nursing administration relevant to designing, planning, and producing nursing for patient populations.

References

Allison, S. E. (1977). Report to the Alumni Association of the Johns Hopkins Hospital School of Nursing on the feasibility study for a practitioner-scholar program for baccalaureate graduates. *Alumni Magazine: Vigilando, 76*(2), 43-58.

Barnard, C. (1962). *The functions of the executive.* Cambridge, MA: Harvard University Press.

Barnum, B. S., & Kerfoot, K. M. (1995). *The nurse as executive* (4th ed.). Gaithersburg, MD: Aspen.

Haynor, P. M. (1996, Summer). Revisioning graduate education in nursing administration: Preparation for a new paradigm. *Nursing Administration Quarterly, 20,* 59-70.

Nyberg, J. (1990). Theoretic explorations of human care and economics: Foundations of nursing administration practice. *Advances in Nursing Science, 13*(1), 74-84.

Orem, D. E. (1989). Nursing administration: A theoretical approach. In B. Henry, C. Arndt, M. Di Vincenti, & A. Marriner-Toomey (Eds.), *Dimensions of nursing administration: Theory, research, education, and practice.* Boston: Blackwell.

Orem, D. E. (1995). *Nursing: Concepts of practice* (5th ed.). St. Louis, MO: Mosby-Year Book.

Senge, P. M. (1990). *The fifth discipline: The art and science of the learning organization.* New York: Doubleday.

Shortell, S. M., Gillies, R. R., Anderson, D. A., Erickson, K. M., & Mitchell, J. G. (1996). *Remaking health care in America: Building organized delivery systems.* San Francisco: Jossey-Bass.

Describing Populations for Purposes of Providing Nursing Services

In this chapter, the process for defining populations requiring health care services is described, with a detailed section on further defining those populations for purposes of planning delivery of nursing services. Building on the variables identified in Chapter 2 as being of concern to nursing, a structure for categorizing information in relation to the nursing perspective of populations is provided, with examples of use of the structure. Defining populations facilitates understanding the requirements for nursing, contributes to identifying the research needs, facilitates developing a documentation system, facilitates developing standards and identifying the skills necessary to provide the nursing service to the population being served, and aids in determining resources required and resource allocation.

General Features of Populations

Studies to determine needs for health care services indicate that the general features of populations addressed include age, gender, morbidity, mortality, and other health-related and sociodemographic variables (Marmor, Barer, & Evans,

1994). As an example of the variety of features of populations studied, a report of the Saskatoon District Health Board Community Development Team (1993) indicated that the following activities related to needs assessment were going on at the same time in that community of approximately 225,000 people:

1. Collection of sociodemographic information by neighborhood
2. Door-to-door survey about leisure activities
3. Study on sexual abuse by Health and Welfare Canada
4. Socio-health survey sponsored by the Red Cross
5. 18 community forums sponsored by the Healthy Saskatoon Project
6. Consultations on poverty
7. Issue-related needs assessment

In addition, statistical databases were being compiled by both the federal and provincial governments, including statistical databases about demographics, economics, and use of health services resources. As a result, health-related problems can be described from a variety of perspectives with some statistics to provide indicators to establish priorities for resource allocation and design of services. For the most part, these data sources fail to include information about the capabilities associated with self-care practices, the exercise of those capabilities, and the impact of factors that condition the development and exercise of those capabilities. The missing variables are in part those that indicate a need for nursing. Because the variables are omitted, planners resort to inferring needs for nursing services from data specific to other health care services, particularly medicine or epidemiology. The necessary information is missing partly because nursing has not been specific in identifying the variables that indicate a need for nursing and ensuring that the data are included in the databases.

Nursing Administration and Population Descriptions

The Utility of Population Descriptions

One of the functions of nursing administration is to initiate and maintain descriptions of populations requiring nursing. These descriptions make it possible for administrators to answer questions about the quality and amount of nursing required over time and at a particular point in time. Population descriptions should also be useful to the administrator in determining the demands that will be placed on nurses in providing the required service. It is not enough to describe populations as those at risk for developing certain health deviations or to refer to obstetrical patients or to medical patients. When these descriptions are used, the need for nursing can only be inferred in a general way. If health care planning is to be comprehensive and include delivery of nursing services, the nursing service requirements must be specified. This requires a basis for specifying the proper object of the service, differentiating nursing from other health professions, and specifying the difference that delivery of such a service should make.

Clinical Data, Nursing Theory, and Population Descriptions

To describe a population, the nursing administrator requires information about preventive health care, medical diagnosis and treatment, prevalence of illnesses in the community, prevalence of injuries, major causes of death, and the health care system, all in order to identify the links between these variables and the self-care practices of persons of concern. This in turn provides direction for development of nursing services. Describing a subpopulation for purposes of developing nursing programs is an iterative process. Information about the population is collected, characteristics are categorized, data are analyzed and descriptions developed, more data are assembled in reference to the categories identified, and further categorization may be done.

Nursing theory can be useful in developing the structure for such data collection and categorization. A comprehensive listing of data items to be considered and a proposed structure for categorizing the data are laid out in Appendix 4A. The data items, derived from self-care deficit nursing theory (Orem, 1995), represent a further elaboration of the variables identified in Figure 2.4. Included are basic conditioning factors, which influence the actions that a person must take to promote or to maintain health and well-being; the therapeutic self-care demand, which provides information about specific purposes of self-care action, such as maintaining a sufficient intake of food; self-care agency, which refers to capability to take the required actions and foundational capabilities and dispositions that are associated with deliberate action; and dependent care agency, which is capability to provide care for a socially dependent person. Needless to say, data about all of the items identified will not be available or necessary in any one situation. Administrators must make judgments about what is necessary.

Case Studies Illustrating Descriptions
of Populations for Nursing Administration Purposes

Two case studies are presented that demonstrate the utility of using the structure for categorizing data to develop population descriptions for nursing administration purposes. The first case study illustrates how the examination of the focus of concern of nurses and the description of nurse activities with individual patients could be used to move from characteristics of individual cases to a different understanding of the nature of the nursing services being provided and required by this subpopulation. The second case study illustrates how the description of a nursing role moved from providing services in relation to specific medical diagnoses to a broader perspective of providing services in relation to self-management systems.

Case 1: Community Health Nurses Describe
a Subpopulation for Nursing Purposes

In the case in point, the law required that persons with tuberculosis were to cooperate with treatment. If not, these persons could be incarcerated in a special ward at one of the hospitals in the community. One role of community health nurses was to follow persons with tuberculosis to ensure that they were cooperating with the prescribed treatment. Working with persons who were alcohol and drug abusers as well as having tuberculosis presented special challenges to the health department. The nurses knew that they were doing more than administering medications and following up on contacts. Their interest in studying this client population in more depth was stimulated when they had some university nursing students assigned to work with them. The students thought nutrition was important: This group of people were not eating properly and should be taught what to eat. But because the persons in question often did not have cooking facilities, teaching what to eat did not seem to be a terribly practical approach.

The community health nurses looked at the characteristics of this population and the kinds of services they were providing to gain some perspective about the characteristics of the client group other than that they were substance-abusing, undernourished persons with tuberculosis who lived in substandard housing and were generally dependent on welfare for financial support. In analyzing what they knew from day-to-day experiences, they identified basically three categories of persons:

1. Older men who lived relatively stable lives. They tended to eat at the same food lines every day, drink in the same bars, and live in the same roominghouse for at least a month at a time.

2. Younger men who were drug as well as alcohol abusers and were much more erratic in their daily living as a result. They were not as regular in the places that they ate and drank and posed a greater problem in terms of treatment and follow-up because it was hard to track them down. However, they still depended on food lines.

3. Young women who often were dependent on men for support and companionship. Their residence varied with the men they were living with, but they too were dependent on food lines.

Analyzing what they knew about the clients further, and with the help of a consultant familiar with nursing theory, they were able to structure the data they had to provide meaningful information about the subpopulation.

They concluded that development of appropriate self-management systems was hindered by lack of knowledge about appropriate health-promoting actions, as well as by certain factors influencing individuals' ability to take appropriate action. Specifically, the conditions of living, lack of adequate resources, results of drug abuse, and sociocultural orientation, among other conditioning factors, interfered with the following:

1. Individuals' ability to consistently act appropriately to manage their self-care

2. The ability to reason within a self-care frame of reference

3. The motivation for self-care

4. The ability to make decisions about care of self and to operationalize these decisions

5. The ability to acquire technical knowledge about self-care from authoritative sources, to retain it, and to operationalize it

On the basis of this analysis and their conclusions, construction of a data collection tool that identified what the specific client population needed to do to promote health and well-being and their capabilities to take appropriate action provided the nurses with ongoing information about changes over time about these elements. Rather than just recording physical findings and medication administration, nurses began to collect data about the health-related management of self-care systems of the population and the factors interfering with that self-management. A different picture of this subpopulation being served by nursing was available for program planning.

For example, in terms of program planning, it became obvious that action was required at the community level for this group of people to meet their requirement to maintain an adequate intake of food. Teaching about what food to eat, how to shop on a budget, and how to prepare food was not an appropriate intervention. These people for the most part did not have access to kitchens or adequate places to store food. Stability of residence was considered to be 1 month! Because they ate at the food lines, action was required to ensure that the food served was such that the requisite related to intake of food would be met.

During the process of developing the data collection tool, it became apparent that nurses were very familiar with the role of nurse as teacher but did not have a consistent way of approaching assessment of capabilities related to self-care. This deficiency became the topic of many inservice education sessions and case conferences.

Some areas of inquiry that arose during this project included, "Why are there no older women in this population?" The focus of medicine with this population was the administration of the medications; what should be the focus of nursing, and what tools were necessary to help nurses achieve their purposes?

In terms of resource allocation, by categorizing the nature of the population and attaching some numbers to each category and by recognizing that the unstable young male group would require the most nursing time per client, it would be possible to get some sense of resource allocation over time. A measure of time required before and after instituting the assessment standards and identification of desired outcomes would also be useful in resource allocation decisions. Identifying the extent to which desired outcomes in relation to nursing were being achieved in the population would give program planners some data to decide whether nurses should simply pass out pills and follow up on tuberculosis contacts or whether they should be involved in more extensive health promotion activity.

Case 2: Redefining the Role of Clinical Nurse Specialist:
Moving From Surgical Procedures or Medical Diagnoses
to Variables Indicating the Need for Nursing

Robinson (1986), a clinical nurse specialist in a large acute care setting whose title was "general surgery clinical specialist," kept data on the patients she was consulted about over the period of a year. This nurse was familiar with nursing theory but had not previously used it to structure what she knew about her patient population. Originally she described her patients as

1. Persons with an ostomy requiring colostomy, ileostomy, or urostomy care
2. Persons with bowel or bladder dysfunction requiring incontinence care or an intermittent catheterization program
3. Persons with impaired skin integrity requiring preventive care as well as pressure sore management
4. Persons requiring wound care and drainage management

She kept patient data related to health state, family systems, conditions and patterns of living, what patients needed to do to manage their health state, and their capabilities to do so. As a result of analyzing these data, she was able to write a job description that more accurately described what she was doing. She identified that her primary focus was on self-care demands arising from requisites related to processes of elimination and maintaining skin integrity. Her scope of practice was described as nursing situations in which patients experienced deficits in meeting those requisites. Thus, rather than being a surgical clinical nurse specialist, she viewed herself as a specialist in management of self-care systems related to elimination and skin integrity. She could describe to physicians and nurses exactly the kind of consultation in which she specialized.

However, the contribution to the planning process was even more significant. A nursing clinic for elimination and skin care problems was established in the outpatient department as a result of statistics being kept that resulted in the identification of a subpopulation of a significant size and in need of a particular type of nursing service. In addition, Robinson identified two other problems of significance requiring further research and study in this group. They were

1. A need to study the relationship between the patients' readiness to learn, their energy level, the energy level of the family caregiver, and the complexity of the management system or number of new self-care demands
2. A need to look at management of self-care systems, considering limited community resources available for management of pain of persons with cancer

In addition to providing a clear definition of her role, Robinson suggested that using nursing theory in defining the populations she served resulted in her focusing on self-management systems, identifying areas needing further study to improve patient care, providing insight into needs for staff development, and providing a road map for developing guidelines for quality care programs.

Patient Variables of Concern to Nursing

The case studies presented above have demonstrated that nursing is concerned with helping patients to develop appropriate management systems for self-care or for providing that care when they are unable to do so. It is concerned with identifying appropriate actions to be taken to promote health and well-being and the capability of the patient to take that action. The process of analyzing what nurses attend to in a patient situation results in identification of the variables of concern to nursing. Specifying these variables and developing operational definitions facilitates collecting data indicative of the needs for nursing in society.

The American Nurses Association (1994), in its social policy statement, referred to the phenomena of concern to nursing as "human experiences and responses to birth, health, illness, and death" (p. 8). Examples identified included care and self-care processes, physiological and pathological processes, comfort, discomfort, emotions, decision-making abilities, perceptual orientations, relationships and role performance, and social policies affecting health. The Nursing Development Conference Group (1979) identified similar phenomena as being within the range of concern to nursing. However, they went a step further in studying the relationships of these phenomena and then formalizing their understanding in a theory of nursing practice—the self-care deficit nursing theory. Formalization of this theory and the subsequent development of the constructs associated with it have provided nursing with the necessary operational definitions of the phenomena or variables of concern to nursing and a means of making the transition from the abstract to the concrete reality of practice.

When a patient population is defined from a nursing perspective, using the variables of concern to nursing as the organizers in that description, as illustrated in the case examples, a view of the population under study with specific reference to nursing and the services it can and should provide emerges. Such an approach also provides additional information about the population and self-care. This type of analysis in relation to health policy formulation, program planning, and decisions concerning resource allocation is necessary to ensure the production of nursing.

Guidelines for Defining a Clinical
Population for Nursing Purposes

As previously indicated and illustrated, the elements and relationships to consider when defining and describing a clinical population for nursing purposes include conditioning factors that are active in the subpopulation, self-care requisites of concern and associated actions required, and types of self-care limitations. A number of cases should be reviewed, identifying the elements that are most significant in relation to the self-care systems of the population under study. After a number of cases have been reviewed, the most commonly recurring variable can be identified, and one or more major organizers emerge. The next step is to establish the range over which the major organizer(s) and other variables that are identified vary for the population. From following this process, a description of the population emerges.

This process is demonstrated in the description in Appendix 4B of a population made up of persons with new spinal cord injuries undergoing initial rehabilitation. The information sources include data from individual cases, experience of nurses working with this group of people, and the literature. The population description is very detailed and was developed for the purpose of designing a nursing system (see Chapter 6 of this book).

Nursing Diagnoses and Defining
Populations for Nursing Purposes

Another means of defining populations of concern to nursing is in reference to nursing diagnoses. Various diagnostic schemas have been proposed; the one most commonly referred to in the literature is that of the North American Nursing Diagnosis Association (Kim, McFarland, & McLane, 1991). Although this schema has been useful for many purposes in nursing, it is not complete or adequate for nurses using self-care deficit nursing theory as a frame of reference for practice. Taylor (1991) proposed a classification system for nursing diagnoses derived from the perspective of self-care deficit nursing theory. The schema presents a means of describing variations in relationships among the patient variables by categories. These categories provide a basis for describing diagnoses at four levels, from the broadest perspective to individual elements. These categories and some examples of constructs within the categories are

1. The whole system in relation to promoting, maintaining, and restoring health and function

2. Major elements—for example, self-care deficits, therapeutic self-care demand, self-care agency
3. Particularistic elements—for example, limitations of knowing, decision making, acting; the power components of self-care agency
4. Most specific elements—the peripheral elements—basic conditioning factors

This classification system can be used to define populations and to describe the specific focus of concern of nursing for program planning. Some examples of subsets of populations that have emerged from use of this diagnostic schema are provided below, along with suggestions for collecting additional data that could be analyzed to provide a more complete picture of the population for nursing purposes.

- Frail elderly, unable to manage self-care because of inability to attend consistently to self as self-care agent. Additional data of interest to nursing would be the age range of the population, most commonly recurring medical diagnoses in this group, incidence of presence of family members who can act as caregivers, conditions of living, patterns of living, and specific self-care requisites most frequently affected.
- Persons needing to develop new self-management systems because of change in health state. Additional data include age range, health state, health care system factors, conditions and patterns of living, self-care limitations and capabilities, and self-care demand.
- Families requiring assistance in meeting family functions with relation to self-care, particularly meeting therapeutic self-care demands of all family members when one member of the family is chronically ill. Additional data would include, for example, age range of family members, health state of affected family member, family system factors, health care system factors, sociocultural factors, and available community resources.

Summary

Administrators of nursing have a responsibility to provide leadership in defining populations requiring nursing and the nature of the services required. It is not enough to describe populations as those at risk for developing certain health deviations or to refer to medical patients or to prenatal clients. When these descriptions are used, the need for nursing can only be inferred in a general way. If health care planning is to be comprehensive and include delivery of nursing services, the nursing service requirements must be more particularly described. In Appendix 4A of this chapter, a structure derived from a comprehensive theory of nursing practice, the self-care deficit nursing theory, is proposed, and its utility for describing populations for nursing purposes is illustrated through case studies and in Appendix 4B.

References

American Nurses Association. (1994). *Nursing's social policy statement.* Kansas City, MO: Author.

Kim, M. J., McFarland, G. K., & McLane, A. M. (1991). *Pocket guide to nursing diagnoses* (2nd ed.). St. Louis, MO: C. V. Mosby.

Marmor, T. R., Barer, M. L., & Evans, R. G. (Eds.). (1994). *Why are some people healthy and others not?* New York: Aldine de Gruyter.

Nursing Development Conference Group. (1979). *Concept formalization in nursing: Process and product* (2nd ed., D. E. Orem, Ed.). Boston: Little, Brown.

Orem, D. E. (1995). *Nursing: Concepts of practice* (5th ed.). St. Louis, MO: Mosby-Year Book.

Robinson, V. (1986). Relationship of theory based nursing and defined populations in practice. In S. G. Taylor (Ed.), *Theory based nursing process and product* (pp. 53-62). Columbia, MO: University of Missouri.

Saskatoon District Health Board Community Development Team. (1993). *Community health needs assessment.* Unpublished working paper.

Taylor, S. G. (1991). The structure of nursing diagnosis from Orem's theory. *Nursing Science Quarterly, 4,* 24-32.

A Structure for Categorizing Data in Describing a Population for Nursing Purposes

1. Basic Conditioning Factors
    1.1. Personal
        1.1.1. Age
        1.1.2. Sex
        1.1.3. Residence and environmental factors
        1.1.4. Family system factors
        1.1.5. Sociocultural factors, including education, occupation
        1.1.6. Socioeconomic factors
    1.2. Patterns of living
    1.3. Health state and health care system factors
        1.3.1. Medical diagnosis
        1.3.2. Nurse-determined conditions

SOURCE: Derived from Orem (1995).

1.3.3. Patient's description of health state

1.3.4. Family member's description of health state

1.3.5. Health care system features—disciplines, services/care

1.4. Developmental state in relation to meeting developmental self-care requisites

    1.4.1. Patient's goals and view of future

    1.4.2. Objective appraisals of developmental potential

    1.4.3. Self-management capabilities considering health state, conditions of living

    1.4.4. Factors necessary for/adversely affecting self-management

2. Therapeutic Self-Care Demand

2.1. Actions associated with universal self-care requisites

    2.1.1. Maintenance of a sufficient intake of air

    2.1.2. Maintenance of a sufficient intake of water

    2.1.3. Maintenance of a sufficient intake of food

    2.1.4. Provision of care associated with elimination processes and excrements

    2.1.5. Maintenance of a balance between activity and rest

    2.1.6. Maintenance of a balance between solitude and social interaction

    2.1.7. Prevention of hazards to human life, human functioning, and human well-being

    2.1.8. Promotion of human functioning and development within social groups in accord with human potential, known human limitations, and the human desire to be normal

2.2. Developmental self-care requisites

    2.2.1. Provide and maintain an adequacy of materials (e.g., water and food) and conditions essential for development of the human body at stages when foundations for bodily features are laid down and dynamic developments occur

2.2.2. Provide and maintain physical, environmental, and social conditions that ensure feelings of comfort and safety, the sense of being close to another, and the sense of being cared for

2.2.3. Provide and maintain conditions that prevent both sensory deprivation and sensory overload

2.2.4. Provide and maintain conditions that promote and sustain affective and cognitional development

2.2.5. Provide conditions and experiences to facilitate beginning and advanced skill development essential for life in society, including intellectual, practical, interactional, and social skills

2.2.6. Provide conditions and experiences to foster awareness of possessing a self and of being a person within the world of the family and community

2.2.7. Regulate the physical, biological, and social environment to prevent development of state of fear, anger, or anxiety

2.3. Health deviation self-care requisites

2.3.1. Seeking and securing appropriate medical assistance

2.3.2. Being aware of and attending to the effects and results of pathologic conditions and states, including effects on development

2.3.3. Effectively carrying out medically prescribed diagnostic, therapeutic, and rehabilitative measures

2.3.4. Being aware of and attending to or regulating the discomforting or deleterious effects of medical care measures performed or prescribed by the physician, including effects on development

2.3.5. Modifying the self-concept (and self-image) in accepting oneself as being in a particular state of health and in need of specific forms of health care

2.3.6. Learning to live with the effects of pathologic conditions and states and the effects of medical

diagnostic and treatment measures in a lifestyle that
promotes continued personal development

3. Self-Care Agency

  3.1. Self-care limitations, capabilities

    3.1.1. Knowing

    3.1.2. Decision making

    3.1.3. Performing self-care

  3.2. Power components of self-care agency

    3.2.1. Ability to maintain attention and requisite vigilance
    with respect to self as to conditions significant for
    self-care

    3.2.2. Controlled use of physical energy for self-care

    3.2.3. Ability to control the position of the body and body
    parts for self-care

    3.2.4. Ability to reason within self-care frame of reference

    3.2.5. Motivation for self-care

    3.2.6. Ability to make decisions about care of self and to
    operationalize these decisions

    3.2.7. Ability to acquire technical knowledge about self-care
    from authoritative sources, to retain it, and to
    operationalize it

    3.2.8. A repertoire of cognitive, perceptual, manipulative,
    communication, and interpersonal skills adapted to the
    performance of self-care operations

    3.2.9. Ability to order discrete self-care actions or action
    systems into relationships with prior and subsequent
    actions toward the final achievement of regulatory
    goals of self-care

    3.2.10. Ability to consistently perform self-care operations,
    integrating them with relevant aspects of personal,
    family, and community living

4. Dependent Care Agency

  4.1. Dependent care capabilities and limitations

    4.1.1. Knowing

4.1.2. Decision making

4.1.3. Producing dependent care

4.2. Power components of dependent care agency

5. Foundational Capabilities and Dispositions

5.1. Conditioning factors and states affecting capabilities and dispositions

5.1.1. Genetic and constitutional factors

5.1.2. Arousal state

5.1.3. Social organization

5.1.4. Culture

5.1.5. Experience

5.2. Selected basic capabilities

5.2.1. Sensation—proprioception and exteroception

5.2.2. Learning

5.2.3. Exercise or work

5.2.4. Regulation of the position and movement of the body/parts

5.2.5. Attention

5.2.6. Perception

5.2.7. Memory

5.2.8. Central regulation of motivational, emotional processes

5.3. Knowing and doing capabilities

5.3.1. Rational agency

5.3.2. Operational knowing

5.3.3. Learned skills—reading, counting, writing, manual, reasoning, verbal, perceptual

5.3.4. Self-consistency in knowing and doing

5.4. Dispositions affecting goals sought

5.4.1. Self-understanding

5.4.2. Self-awareness

5.4.3. Self-concept

5.4.4. Self-value

      5.4.5. Self-acceptance

      5.4.6. Self-concern

      5.4.7. Acceptance of bodily functions

      5.4.8. Willingness to meet needs of self

      5.4.9. Future directedness

  5.5. Significant orientative capabilities and dispositions

      5.5.1. Orientations to time, health, other persons, events, objects

      5.5.2. Priority system or value hierarchy—moral, economic, aesthetic, material, social

      5.5.3. Interest and concerns

      5.5.4. Habits

      5.5.5. Ability to work with the body and its parts

      5.5.6. Ability to manage self and personal affairs

A Population Description

1. *Basic Conditioning Factors*

A spinal cord injury has major effects and results on integrated functioning of human beings. The basic conditioning factors serve as a guide for describing some of the basic operative influencing factors to be understood and considered in nursing of these patients.

   1.1. Health state: Tetraplegia (quadriplegia) or paraplegia arising from trauma—commonly gunshot wounds or acts of violence, automobile and diving accidents, and neurological diseases. Degree and extent of injury varies with cord level of injury and whether it is complete or incomplete. Patients with injuries at C6 or above and C4-5 may be on mechanical ventilators with tracheostomy, medical complications, etc.

      Generally the health state is good, but some may be debilitated if the injury is long-standing and self-management has been ineffectual. Status may be acute to convalescent. If a new injury, 2 weeks or more, initial rehabilitation is needed. The spine may be stable or unstable, nonsurgical or

AUTHORS' NOTE: From "Structuring Nursing Practice Based on Orem's Theory of Nursing: A Nurse Administrator's Perspective," by S. E. Allison, in *The Art and Science of Self-Care* (Figure 22.2, pp. 231-234), edited by J. Riehl-Sisca, 1985, Norwalk, CT: Appleton-Century-Crofts. Copyright 1985 by Appleton Lange. Adapted with permission.

postoperative with or without complications. If the injury is old (more than 6 months), the spine usually is stable. Initial rehabilitation or additional rehabilitation therapy may be required. Some are treated for complications.

1.2. Developmental state: Age range may be from 18 to 50 years on average; adolescents to adulthood; younger males (the majority) often are risk takers, impulsive.

1.3. Education: Level may range from illiterate through college education.

1.4. Psychological state: Adjustment reflects states of stress concerning loss, usually associated with degree of injury and extent of disability along with fundamental personality. If old injury, may have increased motivation and readiness for learning more.

1.5. Sociocultural factors: Population in this situation generally is rural and urban, nonindustrial, agricultural; black and white; all socioeconomic levels; Protestant majority.

1.6. Economic resources: Limited for long-term care, usually governmental—vocational rehabilitation, Medicaid, Medicare, workers' compensation.

1.7. Family systems: Variable family/significant-other support and stability. Support may occur at any given point after injury from preinjury status.

1.8. Environment: Physical and social varies from unavailable, inaccessible, unaffordable, and indifferent to more accessible and accepting, especially since enactment of the Physical Disabilities Law making public facilities available and accessible. Social understanding and acceptance have increased but are not uniform.

2. *Self-Care Agency*

2.1. Capabilities: Unless acutely ill from complications, will cognitively be able to attend to, participate in, and practice therapeutic measures within physical limitations; can learn to perform new or adjusted self-care measures.

2.2. Limitations:

2.2.1. Movement of body: Paraplegia—has upper extremity movement but lacks knowledge and skill to alter body position and use mobility devices; unable to manage lower body and elimination functions.
Tetraplegia—lower extremities immobile; the ability to move upper extremities, breathe, swallow, cough, talk, and move depends on level and severity of cervical cord injury. Improvement in time for either paraplegics or quadriplegics depends on whether cord injury is complete or incomplete.

2.2.2. Lack of awareness of alterations in body functioning; lack of ability to monitor and regulate health condition and treatment related to spinal cord injury.

2.2.3. Lack of knowledge and skill to adjust prior self-care practices to altered condition and integrate into daily therapeutic regime.

2.2.4. Lack of ability to control and pace activity/rest schedule to prevent or reduce fatigue in relation to decreased energy level.

2.2.5. Variable ability to adjust and accept disability and alterations in body and self-image.

2.2.6. Degree of motivation to learn and exercise self-care varies with sociocultural values, family support systems, personality, and life orientation of individual; some have no perception of need or willingness to acquire new self-care knowledge and skills.

2.2.7. Variations in ability to control behavior to the extent needed for self-care and/or permit others to perform care and to consistently tolerate constraints of rehabilitation regimen; difficulty in adjusting to need for and services of dependent care agent (for some tetraplegics).

2.2.8. Extent of development of previous self-care system varies depending on age, values, and interests, sociocultural orientation, and past life experiences as affected by the spinal cord injury. Adolescents' self-care agency is developing, may not be operative, may be inadequate to partially adequate. Adults' self-care agency is developed; not operative to partially operative; inadequate to partially adequate.

2.2.9. Ability to integrate self-care/dependent care with other aspects of daily living; initially may be inadequate.

3. *Dependent Care Agency*

3.1. Dependent care agent limitations: lack of knowledge and skill, willingness, and/or ability to assume the added responsibility and work required to assist another with self-care on a continuing daily basis for life; some lack the physical strength and stamina for this, especially older persons. Frequently, there is despair and resentment about maintaining the dependent at home or returning home on a permanent basis, some of which may be the economic burden of supplies, etc. Some have no one to assume this role and must employ a caregiver.

4. *Self-Care Requisites and Therapeutic Self-Care Demand: Health Deviation, Universal, and Developmental*

4.1. Learn to manage health deviation self-care to:

4.1.1. Become aware of and monitor effects and results of spinal cord injury and treatment on self and body functioning.

4.1.2. Seek and cooperate with medical, nursing, and other therapies and diagnostic measures; follow schedule and practice prescribed measures; assert self in dealing with caregivers; make choices and decisions in planning care.

4.1.3. Become informed about, seek, and use available health care services and resources of the rehabilitation center (chaplain, psychologist, social worker, vocational rehabilitation, etc.) to overcome obstacles to self-care and integrated functioning.

4.1.4. Acquire new knowledge and skills needed to monitor, prevent, and/or manage disability, other existing or potential health problems, medications and treatments required (e.g., dysreflexia, urinary tract infection, skin breakdown, pain, spine instability, gastrointestinal problems, altered sexual functioning, bracing and splints of body parts, and use of equipment).

4.1.5. Adjust or learn to live with alterations in body functioning and body image as affected by changes in sensation, perception, proprioception, self-image, and self-esteem; manage stress associated with injury and demands of health care environment.

4.1.6. On inpatient admission, learn physical environment, routines, rules and regulations of residence, and operation of health care system as different from acute care institution; adjust to living with other patients and staff for extended period of time.

4.1.7. Determine and seek resources to overcome obstacles to self-care at home and in the community—financial, physical equipment, supplies, personal assistance, and alterations in home (ramps, doors, bath, etc.).

4.2. Adjust and manage universal and developmental self-care requisites as altered by spinal cord injury:

4.2.1. Monitor self in terms of new norms in body function and effectiveness of self-care measures to manage:

4.2.1.1. Breathing, coughing, use of respirators and ventilation devices

4.2.1.2. Elimination—bowel and bladder and complications, bathing

4.2.1.3. Nutrition and hydration; eating techniques

4.2.1.4. Mobility measures, prevention of pressure sores, contractures and heterotopic ossification, control of spasticity, range-of-motion exercises

4.2.1.5. Infection—prevent, detect, and treat pulmonary, genitourinary, skin infections

4.2.1.6. Prevention of hazards—fractures, burns, skin trauma

4.2.1.7. Temperature regulation—clothing and protective measures

4.2.1.8. Altered sexual functioning

4.2.2. Manage regimen to control above and engage in activities of daily living using special assistive equipment—wheelchair, commode chair, etc.

4.2.3. Make decisions and choices about schedule of activities; pace self to conserve energy, prevent fatigue, and optimize strength; participate in social activities and rest as needed.

4.2.4. Adjust/revise previous self-care knowledge and practices in relation to new demands and self-care limitations.

4.2.5. Develop and/or adjust self-care system to be compatible with lifestyle and family system in living.

4.2.6. Accept, cooperate with, and/or directly manage care by dependent care agent.

4.2.7. Continue normal development adjusted to disability with relation to sexuality, social roles, family life, educational/occupational, and personal aspirations, beliefs, and activities.

4.2.8. Acquire new living skills, problem-solve, make adjustments and decisions about how to deal with living environment—to physically and socially negotiate in community.

The Processes of Administration

Two foundational organizational documents are the mission and philosophy statements. Clarification of the purposes and goals of nursing on the basis of the self-care deficit theory of nursing in relation to these documents provides direction for structuring the nursing organization and its processes. Critical to all of this is the role and function of the nurse administrator as the leader responsible for the development and maintenance of the nursing focus in the nursing organization and in its processes.

Processes of Nursing Administration

Structuring for Goal Achievement

The structuring of the nursing organization for goal achievement can be understood both as structuring of nursing practice itself based on a theory of nursing and as structuring of the nursing organization for theory-based nursing—establishment and maintenance of the types and numbers of nursing personnel and the interpersonal relationships needed in the organization of nurses to support the provision of nursing. In the first type of structuring, the theoretical nursing framework sets the focus and domain of nursing practice in

85

the policies and procedures, the communication systems, and so forth. In the second, from descriptions of the patient population and subpopulations to be served, production design models can be developed for nursing practice (see Chapter 4 of this book), and appropriate organizational structures can be established to ensure that the production of systems of nursing as designed is carried out. These designs are the basis for developing practice models for nursing caseloads of patients and collaborative practice models for teams of nursing personnel and for multidisciplinary health care teams that include nurses—a current trend. Modes selected for delivery of nursing—team, primary, total patient care—will depend on patient requirements for nursing and available resources of the professional and nonprofessional nursing personnel. The mode of delivery used should take into consideration the number, types, and capabilities of the nurses, the number and complexity of the patients' problems, and many other factors.

Flexibility to adapt to rapid changes in the health care field is a primary concern when structuring nursing organizations to provide nursing. Clarity in the nursing focus—knowing the specific potential contribution of nursing to the populations to be served—provides direction for ascertaining goal achievement and for structuring the organization and processes of practice. An organizational first step is establishment of the mission of the enterprise as a whole. When approved by the governing body, this becomes a guide for designing, developing, organizing, and managing the enterprise. In recent years, employees of many organizations have frequently participated in formalizing the mission statement. Employee involvement is seen as a means to gain commitment to the vision and purposes of the organization. Participation of nursing management in this activity is particularly important if nursing is a major service provided by the organization. Premises set forth in the mission statement should be carried forward in statements of philosophy, operational policies and procedures, and the structure of the organization.

Policy Making

The governing body establishes broad policies for regulating the relations, operations, and outcomes in a health care enterprise. Policies are needed to guide actions in given sets of circumstances. They serve to delineate responsibilities and authority at all levels for various activities in the organization and provide guidelines for safe, effective care of the populations served or to be served. Whether written or unwritten, policies are a form of communication that facilitate decision making and work operations. People know what is expected, how to behave or conduct affairs, and to whom responsibilities and activities are designated. Policy at the executive and operational levels of the organization as derived from the governing board is developed to meet the needs and functions of each organizational unit. The policies and procedures are evaluated and revised as needed by management or by management and the workers together. The aim should be to serve the best interests of the enterprise and all who work within it to ensure provision of the best health care services possible to the patients/clients served. Effort should always be made for continuous improvement as circumstances change and needs arise.

The Mission Statement

A mission statement essentially sets forth the organization's beliefs, goals, and purposes for existence. It may be simply or elaborately stated. The mission statement in part may be derived from statements in the charter of the institution or some other legal document used to establish the enterprise. In a religious institution, for example, the mission statement might incorporate the types of services offered to society in a manner that exemplifies the beliefs of the particular faith. Other organizations may emphasize democratic social ideals in their mission statements along with the purpose(s) and goals of the institution and how the organization hopes to achieve its vision in meeting particular needs in society. Words such as *charitable, caring,* and *provision of high-quality care* (to all or a particular group in the community), and possibly something about cost-effectiveness, may be written into the mission statements. The latter consideration may relate to cost benefits or profit for the institution and/or for the population(s) served. The statement should be sincere and realistic enough to provide meaningful direction for other organizational documents, structures, functions, and operations.

A sample mission statement for a rehabilitation hospital might be as follows:

> (Name of institution) is committed to excellence and leadership in providing comprehensive rehabilitation services and compassionate care to physically challenged individuals and their families for the purposes of helping them to rebuild and enhance the quality of their lives.

Additional statements might include a list of intentions, such as (a) patients and families are the focus of care; (b) the worth and dignity of the individual are promoted; (c) learning opportunities are provided to increase the capabilities and growth of patients, families, and staff; (d) effort will be directed toward creating innovative and effective methods and approaches to care through research and development; and (e) educational programs on rehabilitation for professionals and the community will be offered.

According to Heskett (1986), the mission statement of a health care enterprise should set forth "the strategic vision." It is the logically organized plan for implementing ideas and achieving the target(s) of the enterprise. Senge (1990), the originator of the idea of "the learning organization," carried this further by emphasizing the need to build what he called a "shared vision" such that workers have a vested interest in the vision and a commitment to it. The vision is based on a mental model of what is desired and requires disciplined learning to shed old mental models and work with the new. Personal mastery of the vision, team learning, and systems thinking all are needed to bring the new mental model, the "shared vision," into reality.

Philosophy Statement

Each department in a service organization has written policies. Generally, for professional departments, a statement of philosophy sets forth the beliefs and understandings of a particular discipline, such as nursing, in relation to the mission statement of the health care enterprise. Philosophy statements should serve as guides for practice and organization for delivery of nursing. The question is: How realistic and useful are these statements in terms of providing a solid basis on which to structure, develop, and improve nursing practice? A clear theoretical focus for "thinking nursing"—a mental model—can answer this question. In short, use of a formalized comprehensive theory of nursing, such as the self-care deficit theory of nursing, is the way to put nursing back into nursing administration (Allison, McLaughlin, & Walker, 1991).

Too often, philosophy statements of departments of nursing written in broad, general terms sound good but remain simply words on paper. Nursing is not defined, and the statements lack a sufficient substantive foundation to guide nursing practice and to facilitate the design and development of nursing practice systems as innovative, cost-effective, and efficient services.

Knowing the content of nursing based on the self-care deficit theory of nursing helps nurses to "think nursing" and enables nurse administrators to sort out nursing elements from other dimensions of practice and nursing administration. A number of these factors described as follows can be identified and clarified through the nursing philosophy statements.

■ *Theory as Content Distinguished*
  From Other Dimensions

The theoretical substantive structure of nursing is the central core of nursing practice from which other dimensions in the management of practice can be differentiated. Manthey (1991) referred to professional practice as that over which the nurse exercises control in decision making. Manthey's model for professional practice consisted of four main components: philosophy of management, delivery system, nurse's role, and practice expectations. In the last component, three nursing theorists (theories) and managed care were cited together.

Although Manthey included managed care as part of the theoretical domain over which nursing exercises control in decision making, managed care as described in the literature is not based on a nursing theory. It is a management concept that has been defined in two ways. It is most commonly understood to mean "a set of standardized techniques used by or on behalf of purchasers of health care benefits to manage health care costs by influencing patient decision making through case assistants of the appropriateness of care *prior* [italics added] to its provision" (Powell, 1996, p. 4). But it can also refer to clinical paths or care maps as project management strategies that delineate standardized care in time phases for efficiency of operation, a cost consideration. Clinical pathways may be medically oriented. Nursing goals and processes may not be clearly delineated. Managed care and clinical care paths are not inconsistent with theory-based nursing practice. They are another example of using management and medical orientations to make nursing decisions rather than allowing nursing theory to provide the required direction. Care maps should specify nursing actions to be taken in relation to a range of patient actions or inactions and the self-care deficits and limitations expected at different points on a time line in the process of care. Self-care deficit nursing theory can provide the structure for design of these systems (see Chapters 3 and 4 of this book).

■ *What a Nursing Theory Does*

Nursing theory, then, delineates the substantive structure of nursing—what nursing practice is all about. In writing nursing philosophy statements and in the practice of nursing, knowing the substantive nature of nursing helps to distinguish between (a) the nursing process as theory, (b) problems identified in the National Association of Nursing Diagnosis Association (NANDA) list of diagnoses (NANDA, 1989), (c) the mode of delivery of nursing, and (d) forms of governance in nursing.

The "nursing process" as usually described is simply a problem-solving process applicable to all practice disciplines. Such a process is concerned with actions to solve particular types of problems—diagnosis, prescription, and implementation of interventions or technologies used to solve the problems in light of particular and general goals sought. It includes evaluation of the results obtained and the processes to attain them. The *content* of the nursing process is derived from the nursing theory that is directing the process. In other words, nursing theory becomes the basis for understanding and determining the *nature* of the problem, what the nursing problem is, what is to be diagnosed. For example, from the self-care deficit nursing theory perspective, the problems are the self-care deficits (actual and potential), the limitations in self-care agency, and the basic conditioning factors influencing both.

NANDA provides a list of diagnoses in various categories (Gordon, 1987). From the self-care deficit nursing theory perspective, most are basic conditioning factors or foundational capabilities and dispositions. Included in the list of diagnoses is "self-care deficit." This term as used by NANDA does not have the full range of meaning as defined by Orem. In self-care deficit nursing theory, it encompasses the actions required to meet the universal, developmental, and health deviation self-care requisites in a less-than or negative relationship to self-care agency (persons' self-care abilities and limitations). In NANDA's list, the term *self-care deficit* tends to be interpreted in the more limited sense of personal hygiene. Difficulty arises when nurses try to use both NANDA and the self-care deficit nursing theory at the same time. The NANDA classification does not address the relationship between basic conditioning factors, self-care demand, and self-care agency and is therefore inadequate as a classification of diagnoses for persons using self-care deficit nursing theory. The question remains: What does this mean in terms of the person's self-care system, the therapeutic self-care demand, and associated self-care agency?

The substance of nursing, the content, is what must be delivered as nursing. How nursing is organized to be produced is the mode of delivery of nursing or method of assignment of nursing personnel. It may take a variety of forms, such as primary, team, and functional nursing. Case management is another approach that may include coordination of nursing with other health care services and needed resources within a specific setting or across the continuum of health care—inpatient, ambulatory care, home health, and nursing homes. When the case manager is a nurse, some direct nursing may be given.

TABLE 5.1   Nursing Philosophy Statement

NURSING: The purpose of nursing is to assist the individual to engage in therapeutic self-care (i.e., the health and health-related actions required as inputs to self or environment for the sake of life, health, and effective living) and compensate for inabilities to perform these actions. Nursing assisting actions, therefore, teach, guide, support, and provide a therapeutic environment to overcome self-care deficits—actual or potential—and enhance self-care capacities of individuals (Orem, 1971, 1980). Consequently, the family and/or significant others to the patient are considered as important participating members in the rehabilitation process.

Goals for Nursing:

1. Providing and regulating nursing to ensure achievement of nursing results and efficiency of operation.
2. Promoting professional and occupational development of members of the nursing staff.
3. Managing nursing to maintain its unique contribution to health care including its proper coordination with other health care and hospital services.

SOURCE: From "Philosophy of the Nursing Department," unpublished document of the Department of Nursing, Mississippi Methodist Hospital and Rehabilitation Center, Jackson, MS (1977). Adapted with permission.

In addition, the form of governance of nurses in a nursing department should not be confused with either the substance or content of nursing or the mode of its delivery. "Shared governance" is a form of organization that promotes autonomy and recognition of nurses by seeking to maximize collective participation and collaboration among nurses in managing nursing affairs (Porter-O'Grady & Wilson, 1995). It is an example of the philosophy of management of the organization, whether it is a nursing organization or some other.

■ *Sample Philosophy Statements*

Sample statements extracted from a philosophy of nursing for a rehabilitation hospital where nursing practice was based on the self-care deficit theory of nursing are shown in Table 5.1.

These philosophy statements are in congruence with the aforementioned mission statement for the rehabilitation hospital without repeating specific goals. Note that the statements address what the patient should expect and, specifically, the patient's responsibilities and capabilities for self-care. The purpose of nursing is seen as assisting individuals with self-care. Such statements are more specific than simply saying nursing promotes "quality patient care." A portion of text added later identified general rehabilitation goals and nursing's relationship to them as follows:

The GOALS OF REHABILITATION are directed toward:

1. The person functioning in society;
2. The person as a self-care agent; and
3. The person living within a nursing system, articulated within a dependent care system.

The rehabilitation center later defined *formal object* (focus) of *rehabilitation nursing* as "individuals subject to self-care deficits when biologic events, as a result of internal or external (conditioning) factors, are disruptive to human structural and functional integrity to the extent that integrated functioning is impaired to a greater or lesser degree" (Allison & Guerrant, 1986, n.p.), with the note that "integrated" "refers to man as a rational, biological, psychological, social, and spiritual being" (Orem, 1985, quoted in Allison & Guerrant, 1986, n.p.).

Summary of Structures and Processes Affected

In summary, adoption of the self-care deficit nursing theory framework for nursing practice affects many structures and processes of nursing administration. A conceptual approach to nursing influences educational activities (staff development for nurses to learn the theory and work with it) and management activities (standards of care and practice, the patient classification system based on patient dependency in self-care and acuity, documentation tools, and measurement of nursing outcomes and processes; these are discussed in subsequent chapters). It also can affect recruitment and retention of nurses. When nurses function on a conceptual framework basis, they have a more definite focus and sense of direction. The nurse's role and domain are clarified. Use of a nursing theory, however, does not solve all the problems of nursing, as some nurses may think. Good management, fair personnel policies and practices, and justice in resolving problems continue to be essential.

Nursing Leadership Roles and Functions

Leadership in Nursing

The nurse administrator as the leader in an organization seeks goal attainment by influencing others through interpersonal interactions and communication.

Leadership in nursing is founded on knowing nursing, particularly for the population being served; having a vision about what can and should be done based on a clear mental model or nursing framework; and having current information sufficient to anticipate future needs and possibilities. Leadership is only as effective as it is informed.

Leaders have both the responsibility (obligation to account for one's conduct) and the authority (right to make decisions and take action without higher approval) to expect assent, acceptance, and cooperation of others in achieving the purposes of the enterprise (Gillis, 1994). Leaders set the tone of the environment and help create and maintain the vision, making sure that the mental model in place is operative. Acceptance and use of a nursing theory, for example, depend on the conduct, guidance, and support of the nursing leaders in the situation. These leaders endeavor to counsel, guide, support, and facilitate the efforts of others. Leaders help organize to achieve coordination and collaboration in work effort and seek to obtain needed resources (Griffith, 1995). Leaders act to empower nurses to maximize their capabilities in keeping with the vision and purposes of the organization.

At the present stage of development in nursing, when no one theory of nursing is accepted by all, new nurses employed by an enterprise have a variety of views about what constitutes nursing. Consequently, in enterprises where nursing theory is the foundation for practice, the organization must teach, lead, support, and facilitate all nurses in working with the theory.

Selection of a nursing theory for practice in an enterprise usually is a group process stimulated by the nurse leaders in the organization and/or the nurse administrator. Staff nurses generally are involved in this process. Selection is based not only on adequacy of the theory but on congruence with nurses' beliefs about nursing. Critical to the development of nursing theory in practice is nursing leadership and support, particularly from the nurse administrator. The nursing leader is the one to keep it moving and developing through the many changes and obstacles that may occur in daily operations. The nurse leader must know when to push ahead and when to hold back and wait before moving ahead again, depending on what the nursing staff can tolerate and accept. The nurse administrator may be directly involved in the process or may work through others in leadership roles. But the nurse administrator must always maintain the vision, be supportive of the nurses' efforts, and help to make needed resources available.

When a leader leaves a nursing organization, whether it is a service or educational enterprise, too often the mental model or theory on which practice or education is based is gradually abandoned. Without strong nursing leadership, or under new leadership with a different perspective, theory-based nursing will disappear if the theory-based nursing system is not sufficiently well founded and established and if nursing personnel are not fully committed to it. Old habits are too hard to break, and nurses may revert to old patterns or be expected to meet new expectations. Nursing leadership in a nursing organization must help nurses to know and understand their domain of practice if they are to consistently develop and improve that practice on the basis of a theory of nursing.

When a new leader has a different perspective, change is inevitable. Those committed to the theory-based mental model in use can help the new administrator to understand the model and appreciate its benefits. If the nursing system for the patient population based on the model is well enough established, the substance of it should prevail and be adaptable to change.

Communication

The power of leadership derives from the authority of knowledge and the ability of the leader to provide information and communicate it to others so that cooperation and collaboration are achieved. Barnard (1962) stated that persons will accept communication as authoritative when (a) the message is clear and the recipient can and does understand it; (b) the communication is not inconsistent with the purpose of the organization at the time it is made; (c) at that time, the recipient believes it is compatible with his or her personal interests; and (d) he or she is mentally and physically able to comply with it (pp. 163-165). Leaders not only provide information and ensure its transmission to others but must do so before setting the course of action for others to follow. Leaders continually interpret and reinterpret policies, make and modify plans, and take action using both formal communication systems and informal interpersonal channels. The leaders' commitment to the mental model is transmitted both formally and informally, as evidenced by their involvement with the nursing theory in practice serving as role models to others.

For both clinical and administrative purposes, formal written and verbal communications are needed. Written communications consist of the mission and philosophy statements, policies, and procedures. Verbal communications are the directives and explanations given, discussions, conferences, staff meetings held, and so on. For clinical and administrative purposes, communication by nursing management may consist of verbal and written reports about changes in patient status, nursing personnel needed to meet patient needs, and many other factors that may affect nursing administrative decisions. A variety, and today an overwhelming amount, of clinical data are available through use of various monitoring technologies and computer-generated information systems. The problem is to organize this information in some meaningful and usable form for nursing purposes. This is discussed in Chapter 7.

Written and verbal communications about nursing reveal how the nurse thinks about nursing. Communication extends vertically through the organizational hierarchy and also horizontally as more and more nurses work collaboratively with other health care disciplines. Is the information gathered by nurses redundant, similar to that collected by other health care disciplines, or is it clearly identifiable as different but contributory to the whole of the health care process? For example, in rehabilitation, team meetings are held to discuss identified problems from the perspective of each health care discipline. Each one speaks from the definitive vocabulary of that discipline. If nursing has a limited view of self-care as primarily personal hygiene, then reports will cite problems with the bowel, bladder, and skin management rather than using Orem's broader definition of self-care in terms of how the person or dependent care agent manages the self-care system. In short, nurses and nurse leaders must be able to "talk" nursing in the language of nursing in a way meaningful to members of other disciplines as well as to nurses so that all understand nursing.

Facilitation of Nursing

Facilitation of nursing effort is a primary function of a nursing leader and of nursing administration. Both overt and covert (nonverbal) communications are essential to help others to understand, accept, and work with a nursing theory in practice. Coaching and guiding are continuously needed to help nurses function from a theoretical perspective until it becomes a habit. Observing, listening, sharing what is going on in the process of implementing and working with theory-based nursing, and obtaining feedback about processes and results being obtained are all part of facilitation to obtain cooperation and advancement in nursing operations based on the theory. Making a shared vision of nursing a reality takes much time, patience, persistence, and encouragement for nursing personnel to change their previous modes of thinking and functioning. Senge (1990) noted that in a learning organization, "creating meaning and setting priorities are essential" (p. xii). Establishment of the vision and values, dialogue about them, and systems thinking all serve to make an organization dynamic.

Through communication and facilitation of nursing effort, coordination and collaboration are promoted in an organization. This in turn serves to empower nurses to do a better job, learn, recognize their talents, and contribute to the organization. To be empowered, the nurse must have not only knowledge, skills, and experience in nursing but also a sense of his or her own abilities and powers sufficient to be a positive influence on others. The empowered nurse has a sense of direction and purpose as well as confidence in his or her own abilities. Continued learning to promote professional growth and development in use of a nursing theory, reading current literature, and exchanging ideas with others all contribute to the learning process. This is essential if the nurse is to become comfortable and adaptable in working with the theory and in leading others to do likewise so that commonality of focus and nursing outcomes are achieved. Strategies for helping nurses to learn and use the theory are given in Chapter 12.

Considerations in Change

Rapid change is occurring in the health care field. To be prepared to deal with it, the nurse administrator must have a mental model for nursing that provides sufficient structure to meet the needs for the future. To bring about and adjust to change takes informed thinking, a definitive mental model of nursing, ability to make the mental model known, leadership to help others understand and develop it, communication, support, and coordination of effort to ensure its continuance. As nurse administrators deal daily with change, these capabilities must be brought into action to fulfill the role of nursing administrator.

Introduction of one or more dimensions in nursing practice, such as change in the form of governance or delivery of nursing, in addition to a nursing theory can be very complex and can cause considerable confusion, dissatisfaction, and resistance among nursing staff, especially with the many changes now occurring in the health care industry. This is particularly difficult when nursing theory is not commonly perceived or accepted as the basis for the nursing practice and processes and when the relationship among and differences between delivery modes, governance forms, and nursing theory are not clarified. The mental model for nursing, its purpose, and its relationship to the purpose(s) of the organization provide a clear guide for a nursing organization and for design and planning for nursing practice systems.

Summary

The process of nursing administration begins with the nursing leader in establishing the goals and direction for the organization based on a mental model for nursing. The mental model must be congruent with the mission of the organization and be reflected in the philosophy of nursing and the conduct of the nursing leader and of the members of the organization. How the theory of nursing is reflected in the operations of the organization is explored in subsequent chapters.

References

Allison, S. E. (1977). Report to the Alumni Association of the Johns Hopkins Hospital School of Nursing on the feasibility study for a practitioner-scholar program for baccalaureate graduates. *Alumni Magazine: Vigilando, 76*(2), 43-58.

Allison, S. E., & Guerrant, L. (1986, February 26). *Minutes of MMRC staff conference with Dorothea E. Orem.* Unpublished document, Mississippi Methodist Rehabilitation Hospital and Center, Jackson, MS.

Allison, S. E., McLaughlin, K., & Walker, D. (1991). Nursing theory: A tool to put nursing back into nursing administration. *Nursing Administration Quarterly, 15*(3), 72-78.

Barnard, C. (1962). *The functions of the executive.* Cambridge, MA: Harvard University Press.

Gillis, D. A. (1994). *Nursing management: A systems approach* (3rd ed.). Philadelphia: W. B. Saunders.

Gordon, M. (1987). *Nursing diagnosis: Process and application* (2nd ed.). New York: McGraw-Hill.

Griffith, J. R. (1995). *The well-managed health care organization.* Ann Arbor, MI: AUPHA Press.

Heskett, J. L. (1986). *Managing the service economy.* Boston: Harvard Business School Press.

Manthey, M. (1991). Delivery systems and practice models: A dynamic success in managed care. *Nursing Management, 22*, 28-29.

North American Nursing Diagnosis Association. (1989). *Taxonomy I: Revised 1989.* St. Louis, MO: Author.

Orem, D. E. (1971). *Nursing: Concepts of practice.* New York: McGraw-Hill.

Orem, D. E. (1980). *Nursing: Concepts of practice* (2nd ed.). New York: McGraw-Hill.

Orem, D. E. (1985). *Nursing: Concepts of practice* (3rd ed.). New York: McGraw-Hill.

Porter-O'Grady, T., & Wilson, C. K. (1995). *The leadership revolution in health care: Altering systems, changing behaviors.* Gaithersburg, MD: Aspen.

Powell, S. K. (1996). *Nursing case management: A practical guide to success in managed care.* New York: Lippincott-Raven.

Senge, P. M. (1990). *The fifth discipline: The art and science of the learning organization.* New York: Doubleday.

Design as a Function of the Nursing Professional

Both advanced practitioners of nursing and nurses prepared at the graduate level for administration of nursing services have a significant role in the design of nursing systems for patient populations. It is through design that what is required in the way of nursing is determined on the basis of the characteristics of the patient population. It is also through design that nursing actions to address self-care deficits, limitations in self-care agency, and basic conditioning factors influencing the nursing situation are delineated in an organized way to achieve nursing purposes.

The administrator of nursing and advanced practitioners of nursing collaborate in the design process. From nursing systems designs, the administrator proceeds to estimate the nature and amount of nursing resources needed to produce nursing, plan how nursing will be produced, and manage the production of nursing. Although regulation and control of nursing overall is the responsibility of nursing administration at whatever level of the organization it may be, the advanced practitioner and nurse administrator collaborate in evaluating both the process of delivery and the service product—the outcomes of nursing—to ensure the safety, effectiveness, and efficiency of nursing services.

Design as a function of the professional is not as clearly recognized or understood in nursing as it is in disciplines making a material product, such as a house, car, boat, or work of art. This chapter explores the meaning of design in nursing and the characteristics of design. Some characteristics of design and some examples of design for patient populations in various situations are presented.

Meaning of Design

To construct or make something, a design or pattern is needed. A design consists of elements and their associated details laid out in orderly fashion and relationships revealing *what* is to be done. Design precedes a plan because the plan delineates *how* the design is to be implemented and fulfilled. Design is a professional function in practice disciplines such as engineering, architecture, and medicine. For example, a surgeon, drawing on extensive knowledge and experience, determines what procedure is needed and designs or tailors it to meet a particular patient situation. In nursing, design as conceived by Orem (1995) is one of seven professional nursing operations. The social, interpersonal, and technological dimensions (the nursing process components) are outlined in Figure 6.1 in relation to selected elements in the self-care deficit nursing theory. Design involves all of these dimensions.

The notion of design, however, is not generally understood or accepted in nursing because the focus still tends to be on planning for care for individuals, with the planning process combining the "what" and the "how" without differentiating between the two. For nursing, the product of design is a particular type of nursing system—wholly compensatory, partly compensatory, or supportive-educative. The product of nursing is the production of the service—nursing. In the process of implementing the designs for an individual or for a group of individuals, revision or redesign of the whole or some components may be needed due to changes in conditions, outcomes, and goals desired and the emergence of or change in self-care requisites to be met. Continuing diagnosis and prescription of actions to be performed serve to adjust or alter the nursing system.

Generally, a design is understood to be a preliminary outline, an arrangement or drawing, or a pattern. It does not have to be in writing; it may be a mental plan or scheme of approach to doing or making something (*Pocket Oxford Dictionary,* 1984, p. 253). According to the Joint Commission on Accreditation of Healthcare Organizations (1995), design "refers to the rational, deliberate

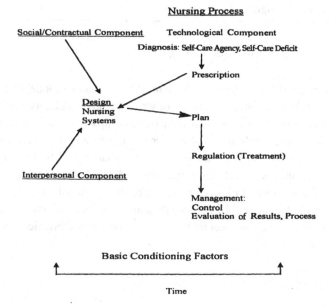

Figure 6.1. Professional Practice Operations

process of creating a quality service as viewed by those who receive it" (p. 39). From a professional practice point of view, the goals of nursing design should go beyond the limitations of a recipient's perspective and seek to achieve definable outcomes of nursing separately and also in conjunction with the contributions of other health team members.

The design of a nursing system, according to Orem (1995), rests on the nurses' knowledge of the work that needs to be done and the relations to be dealt with in doing the work. It must conform with what is needed and what can be done in practice at a particular time and place. The very word *system* implies bringing about or the existence of definable relationships, organization, and order. Design seeks to accomplish harmony and integrity for the system as a whole, for each part or subsystem, and for the relationships between and among the parts and to the whole (Orem, 1995). Nursing system design is very complex. It incorporates the social, interpersonal, and technological dimensions of practice. Factors affecting design include age in relationship to the state of development and engagement in self-management and self-care of adults and children, the health state, the health results sought, the patient/client's point of view, cooperation and coordination, and health care system factors (Orem, 1995).

The Process of Design

Design and a Mental Model of Nursing

To design a nursing system, the nurse must have a mental model of and for nursing, a theoretical conceptualization of what nursing is and what it seeks to achieve. The abstract elements and their relationships in the self-care deficit theory of nursing provide the structure for examining and dealing with real-world situations. The theory variables point to what should be investigated, designed, and planned in relation to the types of nursing results and general health care results desired in concrete situations. In a personal communication, D. E. Orem (1991) stated, "Design is a dynamic process involving movement of thought. Unless one has a feel for the wholeness of clinical practice, one does not understand design."

The Design Units and Their Outcomes

Six parts of a nursing design that Orem (1995) called *design units* are

1. The contract for nursing, concerned with nursing's area of jurisdiction that contributes to the health care goals
2. Establishment of the legitimate and functional unity of care providers
3. Description of components of current or prior self-care or dependent care systems
4. Establishment of the nature of the therapeutic self-care demand and factors that condition those components, including identification of the resources needed to produce nursing and meet the therapeutic self-care demand
5. Establishment of self-care abilities and roles of persons under health care
6. Establishment of the design for the production of nursing by defining role responsibilities for knowing and meeting the therapeutic self-care demand of the persons in the population requiring nursing and the nursing prescriptions for courses of actions—care measures—needed to meet the therapeutic self-care demand and for regulating the person's development or exercise of self-care agency (pp. 255-260)

The design units should identify all the information needed to provide effective nursing. Each unit is and has a general outcome that can be specified concretely (see Table 6.1).

TABLE 6.1 Design Unit Outcomes

Unit	Outcomes
Contract and jurisdiction	Agreement to provide nursing
Legitimate and functional unity	Legitimates situation and participants' responsibility
Self/dependent care	What patients/clients do/have done
Therapeutic self-care demand	Specified self-care actions
Patient/client self-care role	What patients can, should, and should not do
Nursing system design	Production pattern

The problem in design, whether for an individual patient (a nursing case) or for a patient population, is one of attaining desired goals or purposes to maximize results while minimizing and controlling undesired effects or results. In other words, the objective is to bring about the best balance between opposing requirements, avert possible unwanted consequences, and obtain intended results. It frequently is a matter of trial and error (Pye, 1964). Effective design depends on the knowledge, creativity, and skill of the designer.

The Principles of Design

Three broad principles applicable to design of nursing systems are effectiveness, adequacy, and efficiency. The principle of *effectiveness* is concerned with achievement of intended nursing and general health care results. *Adequacy* refers to quality in the sense that the actions are sufficient to the purpose. Four principles of *efficiency* are organization, communication, coordination, and cooperation (D. E. Orem, personal communication, 1991). In addition, three useful principles from industrial engineering particularly pertinent to design for patient populations are specification, standardization, and simplification (Gaither, 1980). Critical pathways or care maps would exemplify this. These three principles are concerned with economy of effort, time, and resources.

Specification of the elements and details for each design unit and how units are organized culminates in the design of the nursing system as a whole. An analogy can be made to an architectural blueprint for construction of a house that lays out the number of floors, the type and number of rooms, and how each element relates to the others to achieve a functional, attractive whole. When a group of houses are to be constructed (or patients to be cared for), the principle of efficiency in use of resources—personnel and time—is particularly relevant.

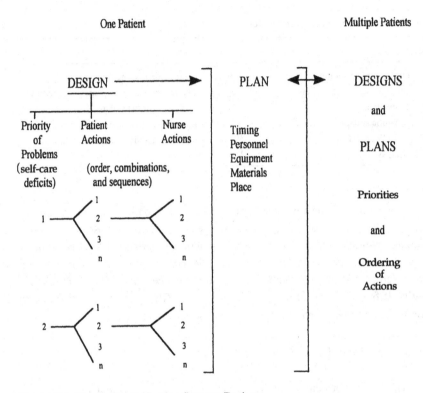

Figure 6.2. Complexity in Nursing Systems Designs

But a house is a concrete entity, not an action system involving interactions of human beings. Standardization and simplification particularly relate to efficiency in design of systems in which different types and numbers of nursing personnel provide care to numbers of patients. A caveat here is not to lose sight of the requirements and desires of individual patients.

The Complexity of Design and Planning for Individual Patients

To obtain a notion of the complexity of design and planning for a specific patient, see Figure 6.2, in which priorities of nursing problems, ordering of patient and nursing actions, and planning as influenced by designs and plans for multiple patients are illustrated.

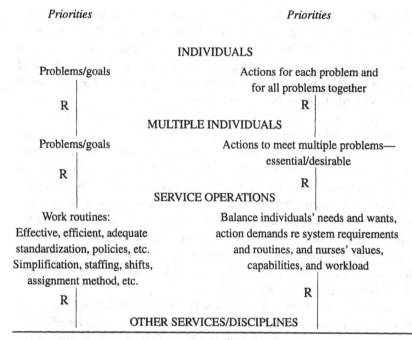

Figure 6.3. Interaction in Nursing Systems Design
NOTE: R = relationship

Interactions in Nursing Systems Designs

In Figure 6.3, the interactions in designs for nursing systems for individual patients, multiple individuals, service operations, and other health care disciplines are further illustrated, showing the number and variety of interactions that must be taken into consideration in nursing systems designs for patient populations.

Issues in Design for Patient Populations

Generalized to a patient population, design of nursing systems is even more complex in terms of the principles of standardization, specification, and simplification. Action sequences to manage one type of problem may also be applicable to others. Designs must be flexible to allow for individual differences and for changes in conditions associated with the patient, the environment, and the providers of nursing. Care maps or critical paths are a form of nursing design only if the specific nursing problems and nursing actions—not just the areas requiring medical monitoring and regulation by nurses—are delineated. General standards of care can be used but should address particular types of nursing problems based on patient limitations in self-care.

For example, in rehabilitation nursing, standards of care relevant to a general case involving self-care include prevention of hazards (e.g., falls and injuries associated with visual and cognitive impairment or impaired mobility), addressing of limitations in communication, addressing of limitations in emotional control, regulation of bowel and bladder function, maintenance of skin integrity, and activities to manage/prevent extension of stroke and hypertension. These standards can be incorporated into general designs of nursing systems for different types of patients but must be particularized to individual situations. Standards such as these help in planning for the provision of nursing utilizing different types and levels of nursing personnel to ensure the availability and effectiveness of the nursing provided.

The validity of nursing systems design is manifested "whenever the design for what is to be produced and what should be" meets the criteria for effectiveness and economy of time and resources (Orem, 1991, p. 115). Skilled design is a creative act, part of the art of nursing.

A number of examples of nursing systems designs for individual patients are to be found in the literature (Clang, 1985; Fawdry, Berry, & Rajacich, 1996; Garritt, 1985; Orem, 1995; Orem & Taylor, 1986). Examples of designs of nursing systems for patient populations based on the self-care deficit nursing theory are more limited (Allison, 1973, 1985; Nursing Development Conference Group, 1979).

Nursing Systems for Patient Populations

When large groups of persons are in need of nursing, design is a means for structuring nursing practice to ensure the availability and provision of nursing to meet the nursing requirements of the patient population served by a health care agency. In recent years, efforts to systematize care provided in acute care institutions have been undertaken in the form of critical paths or care maps. These standardized protocols lay out on a time line the types of care actions to be performed for particular types of patients by a variety of health care personnel, particularly nurses. Critical paths not only delineate steps to be taken in the process of care over time but may include expected outcomes for each phase of care. The Joint Commission standards for accreditation of health care organizations require that the standards be patient centered, multidisciplinary, and organized around the functions common to all health care disciplines in the organization. This does not preclude specifying theory-based nursing standards and outcomes.

An Interdisciplinary View of the Health Care Encounter

Before focusing on design of a nursing system for a population, nursing must be viewed in the context of other disciplines in the health care system because health care is delivered within an interdisciplinary environment. In addition, it also is no longer appropriate to think only of the nursing episode as provided in a particular setting; the nursing needs of a population must be considered across a trajectory of need, including the potential for service delivery for the same encounter to occur in a variety of settings. This trajectory view of an encounter with the health care system has major implications for the communications system. The model in Table 6.2 lays out these factors in the health care flow process from first contact and diagnosis, to implementation of an initial plan of care, through reevaluation of patient family status and a continuing plan of care. In examining this model, note that there is an extreme likelihood that the only person remaining constant throughout the trajectory will be the patient. Though family is listed for each area, there is no certainty that a family member will be present.

The Population Description

Design of a nursing system for a patient population begins with a description of the nursing characteristics of that population (see Chapter 4 of this book). This requires that the nurse administrator know and understand the types of service to be provided by the agency and the consequent demands for nursing based on the number and severity of self-care deficits potentially incurred and the anticipated limitations in self/dependent care agency of the projected population. The nurse administrator must seek and use all available information from a variety of resources in the agency, the community, nursing, and health care in

TABLE 6.2 An Interdisciplinary View of the Health Care Encounter

	Initial Contact		Implementation of Plan of Therapy in First Setting	Reevaluation of Patient/ Dependent Care Agent Status, Diagnoses and Decisions About Therapy/Treatment	
	Diagnosis	Decisions About Therapy		Continue	Discharge
Participants	Family physician Specialist physician Nurse Social worker Therapist Nutritionist Etc.	Initial health care professional Other health care professionals	Physician(s) Nurse(s) Social worker(s) Therapists(s) Nutritionist	Physician(s) Nurse(s) Social worker(s) Therapist(s) Nutritionist	
	PATIENT	PATIENT	PATIENT	PATIENT	PATIENT
	Family	Family	Family	Family	Family
Location	Community		Facility (inpatient) Facility (outpatient) Home Community intervention	Same or new location	Same or new location
Communication system	Demographics Patient characteristics	Health care decision Plan of treatment Contract with patient/family	Tracking of therapy provided Tracking of patient response Tracking of patient/family participation Monitoring of standards/outcomes	Tracking if move, transfer information	Transfer information Maintain record Flag reevaluation

general to aid in designing appropriate, effective, and efficient nursing systems for the patient population. Identification of the general nursing characteristics of a population based on the types of services to be provided, such as acute care, rehabilitation, home care, or hospice, and projection of the predominant self-care requisites and anticipated deficits are needed. Designs of nursing systems for populations should meet a predictable range of nursing requirements of the patient population, yet make allowances for unpredictable events as well.

Use of a Production Model

In Figure 6.4, the elements of a nursing production design model and the relationships among them as derived from Orem's conceptualizations about nursing are laid out in flowchart fashion. The model serves as a guide for designing and planning for the production of nursing for individual nursing cases or a population of patients. It illustrates how variables of concern to nursing identified in Figure 2.4 can be organized for design purposes.

For large groups of persons in need of nursing, the types of nursing problems—the range of self-care requisites to be met and self-care agency potential or lack thereof—need to be identified. From this, the types of nursing systems and types and numbers of nurses needed to produce them can be estimated. The model shows general health goals of life, well-being, and effective living applicable to all health care disciplines and for patients. How self/dependent care and nursing contribute to these goals is shown as results to be achieved. The provision and distribution of nursing services require design, planning for production of nursing, production, and regulation or control of the production of nursing in time and over periods of time. Financing of nursing is based on expenditures for facilities, personnel, resources, time, and the nature of the effort required. Expenses must be controlled in relation to revenues to ensure a viable organization and a reasonable profit margin where profit is the incentive of the organization.

Design Operation and Principles

Table 6.3 shows a simplified model of the components of design based on Orem's self-care deficit nursing theory. It simply outlines how the two design operations of organizing self-care components and selection of ways to meet requirements for care should be consistent with the principles of effectiveness, efficiency, and adequacy as they relate to accomplishing general health goals.

TABLE 6.3 Design Operations and Principles

Operations	Principles	Nursing Goals	Health Goals
Organization of components of therapeutic self-care Selection of a combination of ways of assisting (methods/measures)	Effective Efficient Adequate	Self-care is accomplished Self/dependent care agency is developed/ regulated and protected	Life Health Well-being

Examples of Activities in Nursing Systems Design

Designing a Nursing System for an Inpatient Obstetrical-Gynecological Population

A number of years ago, a project was undertaken to design a nursing system for an inpatient obstetrical-gynecological population. An analysis of admissions data revealed that surgery for myomata uteri was the most common admitting diagnosis. Initial work focused on this to analyze the effects and results on self-care as preliminary to determining the actual design. Flowcharts were developed to analyze each phase and step of the health care encounter. Descriptions of the medical practices were laid out for each phase. The patient population was classified into four broad categories, and specific considerations for each were identified. The categories were

1. Life-giving, life-bearing, and mothering capacities
2. Pathology of genital organs or related supporting structures
3. Pathology of excretory organs
4. Sexual identity and related personality problems

Any number of combinations of these categories might exist (NDCG, 1979).

To examine the contacts that a patient has with various participants in the health care process, Joan Backscheider (1970) developed a flowchart to identify all contacts in the outpatient and inpatient care processes. A portion of this flowchart is reproduced in Figure 6.5. Although the details of the encounter

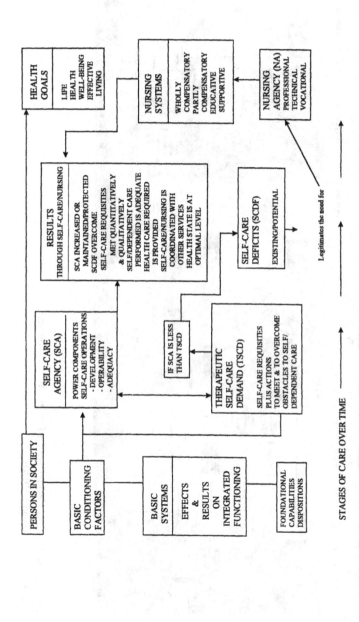

Figure 6.4. Nursing Production Design Model

SOURCE: From "Structuring Nursing Practice Based on Orem's Theory of Nursing: A Nurse Administrator's Perspective," by S. E. Allison, in *The Art and Science of Self-Care* (Figure 22.1), edited by J. Riehl-Sisca, 1985, Norwalk, CT: Appleton-Century-Crofts, Copyright 1985 by Appleton Lange. Adapted with permission.

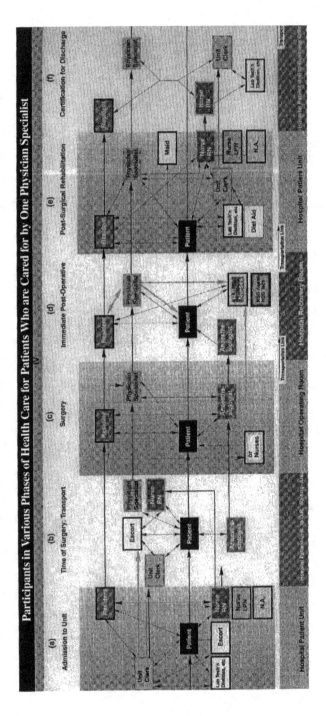

Figure 6.5. Phases of Health Care for Patients With Myomata Uteri
SOURCE: Backscheider (1970).

112

would be different in today's setting, the process of identifying participants is still valid.

Note that the one constant in the care process is the patient! No nurse appears to be consistently in contact with the patient. Nor was there at that time continuity of information flow between outpatient and inpatient services, a problem in some settings today (Renner & Sward, 1997). The phases identified in the flow model served as the basis for developing worksheets preliminary to designing the nursing system, specifically to identify the parts to be addressed. These were

Part I   Health care focus (reason under health care)
Part II   Health deviation self-care related to
           A: Diagnosis and treatment
           B. Adjustments in usual self-care
Part III   Universal self-care
           A. No adjustment to environment
           B. Adjustment to environment
Part IV   Health care judgment concerning given self-care demands
Part V   Nursing requirements
Part VI   Design of nursing system

Designing a Nursing System for a Spinal Cord Injury Population

This framework was adopted by Allison (1985) when analyzing the care requirements and laying out the dimensions of a nursing system for a spinal cord injury population. In Chapter 4, Appendix 4A, a brief description of the patient population in relation to the basic conditioning factors is given, and selected elements of nursing systems are outlined.

In physical rehabilitation, though there may be others, five broad areas of self-care limitations can be identified:

1. Limitations in movement arising from spinal cord injury, brain injury, other neurological impairments, joint replacements, and injury to the musculoskeletal system
2. Limitations in cognitive functioning associated with brain injury
3. Limitations in adaptation of self and lifestyle associated with physical disability
4. Limitations/inability of dependent care agent to accept/manage the dependent's self-care and/or his or her combined self/dependent care systems

TABLE 6.4 Partly Compensatory Nursing Design for a Patient With a Right Cerebrovascular Accident (Immediate Phase of Rehabilitation—Admission, First 48 Hours)

Priority No.	Problem (S-C Deficits/ Limitations	Goals (TSCD Met/S-C Limitations Overcome)	Patient/Family Actions	Nursing Actions
1.	Does not attend to risk for falls/ injuries R/T R CVA	Beginning awareness Accept safety precautions Not remove safety devices	Request help, call nurse Use call light for assistance Patient/family begin to learn risks/need for safety measures	Place bed to observe/monitor qh for needs and safety, right-side orientation Select room near nurses' station Orient to and check use of call system, bed operation Bed check system Posey vest Lap board for wheelchair Supervise/assist with mobility activities Red-flag precautions (back of wheelchair) Instruct patient/family, significant other in safety precautions Teach patient/family safety measures and rehabilitation routines
2.	Lacks new knowledge of equipment/hospital routines R/T limited attention span, unawareness, memory deficit from L hemiparesis	Begin to use equipment appropriately Beginning awareness of daily schedule of times	Use nurse call system Operate bed, TV, etc. Recognize primary nurse	Orient and daily reorient to nurse call, unit therapy schedule, primary nurse, head nurse Explain each activity/task step by step and reinforce positively Establish basic communication system Monitor/validate cognitive functioning/changes Instruct family/significant other in routines/program

3. Unable to communicate appropriately R/T spatial learning limitation affecting perception, naming objects, time/place	Find, name objects appropriately Know schedule, order of activities, time, place	Perform simple tasks Repeat/remember simple object names, schedule Attend/participate in reality orientation classes Follow verbal, visual cues	Break tasks down into simple steps Use pictures/visual cues with printed names as memory aids Give time, repeat, positive reinforcement Schedule reality orientation classes
4. Unaware of left side R/T impaired spatial concepts and decreased awareness of L body parts and placement	Recognize limitation and attend to L side of body	Turn head to see and check L side, feel and find with right side Be aware of total environment Family guide in use of techniques	Locate bed with unaffected side toward door Place objects for orientation to R side Cue to left and look to left often Teach to use R hand to feel, find left side Reassure when agitated Teach techniques to family
5. Limited awareness of behavior changes—impulsiveness, errors, inconsistencies in actions	Become aware, begin control of behavior, correct errors, inconsistencies, etc.	Perform tasks in correct sequences Try to correct errors, cooperate with others	Reduce distractions Focus on one step at a time until tasks are completed Correct errors and behavior promptly Praise, reinforce success Teach techniques to family, seek family cooperation and support
6. Limited ability/unable to control elimination R/T physical limitation above	Control with assistance	Monitor for need/request toileting assistance as needed	Establish toileting program Observe results, adjust Monitor intake/output Monitor/assist with hygiene, skin care, etc. Monitor condition and treatments
7. Lacks new knowledge and skills to manage effects/results of condition/treatments for stroke and hypertension and to adjust universal, developmental system in daily living	Verbalize/demonstrate appropriate care measures Begin to consider developing acceptable design of self/dependent care system to be implemented at home	Participate in individualized and class instruction Practice self/dependent care tasks Learn medications Participate in design of care in hospital and for home	Teach basic techniques and requirements to monitor/manage Consult clinical nurse case manager on specialized individual/group instruction and discharge planning In collaboration with patient and family, begin to explore design of care system for home care/need for home health referral

NOTE: CVA, cerebrovascular accident; L, left; R, right; R/T, related to; S-C, self-care; TSCD, therapeutic self-care demand.

In Appendix 6A, the nursing system for the spinal cord injury patient population described in Chapter 4 is presented. For another less detailed approach to describing a type of nursing system for an ambulatory diabetic patient population, see Allison (1973).

Designing a Nursing System for Patients
With a Right Cerebrovascular Accident

The model of a partly compensatory nursing system shown in Table 6.4 focuses on the immediate phase of rehabilitation. It delineates the components of the nursing process in terms of the diagnosis of the nursing problems (what is and why): new, possibly temporary, and possibly long-term self-care deficits due to limitations in movement and cognitive functioning—left hemiparesis from right cerebrovascular accident. The nursing problems are identified in general order of priority, and prescriptions of nursing actions (what can/should be), the ways of assisting to be performed, are listed in relationship to anticipated patient actions. Note that the types of actions for one type of problem may be applicable to others. The design consists of what will be, in this case, a partly compensatory nursing system. The prognosis is the prediction of the potential outcomes. The person will return home and have a partially operative self-care system within a dependent care system (probably a spouse) under home health care supervision. Each of the broad problems listed can be addressed in specific detail in an actual situation and be adjusted as changes occur. Note that Problem 7 would include all of the self-care requisites and demands that pertain but are not listed here, such as personal hygiene, exercise, intake of food and water, and management of medications. These specifics can be spelled out at a later phase of care.

In this type of nursing case, one type of nursing problem may be closely related to another. Cognitive and visual impairments affect many activities. The order of priority in actions may fluctuate or change with alterations in events or circumstances at any one point in time. Hence, Orem's comment, previously cited, that design must be dynamic and must maintain a view of the whole picture is highly relevant.

In Chapter 7's Appendix 7A, the sample forms "Nursing Action Plan: Immediate" and "Nursing Action Plan: Continuing" operationalize the design function in a rehabilitation population. The action plan form reveals the common areas to be addressed: self-care requisites, the potential nursing goals, the

TABLE 6.5 Designing a Program for Delivery of Nursing Services in Preschool Facilities

---

1. Population of concern: Preschool children in day care facilities
    a. Authority: Criteria for licensing of day care facilities
        (i) Facility and environment
        (ii) Health program
        (iii) Capability of operators to provide care
    b. Desired outcome: a health program for preschool facilities
        (i) Environments that facilitate healthy growth and development of preschool children
        (ii) Caregivers who are able to meet the therapeutic self-care demand of preschool children and thereby contribute to the promotion of life, health, well-being, and development
        (iii) Identification of children with health-related problems that interfere with normal growth, development, and learning
2. Context within which program development occurs (see Appendix 6B for details):
    a. Mission and goals of the city health department
    b. The organizational structure of the city
    c. Philosophy of community health nursing
    d. Standards of nursing practice
3. Role of the nurse
    a. Planning in relation to meeting the health-related needs of the preschooler and facility staff to meet those needs or to access appropriate assistance
    b. Assessment, screening, and referrals
        (i) Primary assessor making appropriate referrals
        (ii) Working with staff of day care
        (iii) Working with parents
    c. Health education
    d. Health promotion
4. Assessment to determine services required in facilities:
    a. Use of assessment standards to determine services required in general facilities
    b. Use of assessment standards to determine services required in special needs facilities
    c. Use of assessment standards to determine adequacy of environment and capability of facility staff to provide health-related care required
5. Collaboration with related disciplines and community agencies/representatives to develop required program:
    a. Services to be provided
    b. Criteria for referral (requirement for assessment/intervention from another perspective)
    c. Definition of roles
    d. Establishment of budget

TABLE 6.5 *(continued)*

6. Unit of service:
   a. Individual child
   b. Individual child and facility staff
   c. Individual child and family member
7. Methods to achieve desired outcomes, including collaboration with related disciplines and community agencies:
   a. Prescribing therapeutic self-care demand (see Appendix 6B)
   b. Inspection and licensing of facilities
   c. Screening on health and developmental state of child
   d. Consultation/advising on:
      (i) Strategies for meeting therapeutic self-care demand of preschool children
      (ii) Promoting self-care skills of children
      (iii) Participation in assessment and screening of preschool children
      (iv) Liaison with and/or development of related community groups and activities

SOURCE: McLaughlin and Walker (1989).

patient/caregiver actions, and nursing actions needed for the initial 48 hours of care. All of these forms are designed to save writing yet allow for individualization according to the patient situation. Other forms in this package are progress notes and a summary form to denote changes/maintenance of status over time at admission and at discharge.

Outline of Program Design in Community

McLaughlin and Walker (1989) used self-care deficit nursing theory for direction when designing the nursing component of a larger community-based program (Table 6.5). Note in this example how the use of the theory gives direction for specifying the focus of nursing in the licensing program for day care facilities. The role of the nurse in relation to the facility staff, the parents, and the children is described. The mental model for the nursing component of the preschool program is the same "mental model" used to develop the standards for nursing practice in the health department. This is an example of the nursing component of the preschool program being an organizational unit within the preschool program at the same time as being a component of the organizational unit of nursing as an entity throughout the enterprise (see Chapter 3). The assessment standards as they have been integrated into the program are one of the means for measuring the effectiveness of the overall program.

Summary

In this chapter, design of nursing systems has been explored and examples have been presented. Design is seen as a particularly important function of the advanced professional practitioner of nursing as the one most clinically knowledgeable about a particular patient population and of nursing administration responsible for ensuring the safe, effective provision of nursing in a cost-effective manner.

References

Allison, S. E. (1973). A framework for nursing action in a nurse-conducted diabetic management clinic. *Journal of Nursing Administration, 3*(4), 53-60.

Allison, S. E. (1985). Structuring nursing practice based on Orem's theory of nursing: A nurse administrator's perspective. In J. Riehl-Sisca (Ed.), *The science and art of self-care* (pp. 225-238). Norwalk, CT: Appleton-Century-Crofts.

Backscheider, J. E. (1970). *Working papers.* Unpublished documents, Woman's Clinic Project, Center for Experimentation and Development in Nursing, Johns Hopkins Hospital, Baltimore.

Clang, E. D. (1985). Nursing systems design for a young married diabetic. In J. Riehl-Sisca (Ed.), *The science and art of self-care* (pp. 113-125). Norwalk, CT: Appleton-Century-Crofts.

Fawdry, M. K., Berry, M. L., & Rajacich, D. (1996). The articulation of nursing systems with dependent care systems of intergenerational caregivers. *Nursing Science Quarterly, 9*(1), 22-26.

Gaither, N. (1980). *Production and operations management.* Hinsdale, IL: Dryden.

Garritt, A. P. (1985). A nursing system for a patient with myocardial infarction. In J. Riehl-Sisca (Ed.), *The science and art of self-care* (pp. 142-169). Norwalk, CT: Appleton-Century-Crofts.

Joint Commission on Accreditation of Healthcare Organizations. (1996). *1996 comprehensive accreditation manual for hospitals.* Oakbrook Terrace, IL: Author.

McLaughlin, K., & Walker, D. (1989, June). *Development of a program for health department services for preschool children in daycare facilities.* Paper presented at the Sixth Annual Institute on Self-Care Deficit Theory, Columbia, MO.

Nursing Development Conference Group. (1979). *Concept formalization in nursing: Process and product* (2nd ed., D. E. Orem, Ed.). Boston: Little, Brown.

Orem, D. E. (1991). *Nursing: Concepts of practice* (4th ed.). St. Louis, MO: Mosby-Year Book.

Orem, D. E. (1995). *Nursing: Concepts of practice* (5th ed.). St. Louis, MO: Mosby-Year Book.

Orem, D. E., & Taylor, S. G. (1986). Orem's general theory of nursing. In P. Winstead-Fry (Ed.), *Case studies in nursing theory* (pp. 59-68). New York: National League for Nursing.

The pocket Oxford dictionary of current English (7th ed.). (1984). New York: Oxford University Press.

Pye, D. (1964). *The nature of design.* New York: Reinhold.

Renner, A., & Sward, J. C. (1997). Patient care data set: Standards for a longitudinal health medical record. *Computers in Nursing, 15*(2), S7-S13.

General Nursing System Design for New Spinal Cord Injury Patients

Factors Affecting Predictability of Outcomes

1. Whether the injury is complete or incomplete
2. Premorbid personality and operability of self-care agency
3. Extent of therapeutic self-care demand in relation to abilities of individual/dependent care agent
4. Socioeconomic-cultural influences on a) adjustment and b) effectiveness of self-management (i.e., when resources—financial, medical, and care provider—are limited, effectiveness of care management is diminished)
5. Time for adjustment—may take 2 to 4 years for both tetraplegics and paraplegics

AUTHORS' NOTE: From "Structuring Nursing Practice Based on Orem's Theory of Nursing: A Nurse Administrator's Perspective," by S. E. Allison, in *The Art and Science of Self-Care* (Figure 22.2, pp. 231-234), edited by J. Riehl-Sisca, 1985, Norwalk, CT: Appleton-Century-Crofts. Copyright 1985 by Appleton/Lange. Adapted with permission.

Types of Nursing Systems Based on Nature and Extent of Self-Care Deficits

Initial Rehabilitation, Tetraplegic

Complete deficits, with the exception that some patients have some knowledge about meaning of the injury to their future and present loss; helplessness requires wholly compensatory nursing system
Goals:

1. Partially compensatory system via dependent care agent by discharge from hospital
2. An educative-supportive nursing system may be needed by individual and dependent care agent on an episodic basis for rest of life
3. Independent with episodic ambulatory care services as needed

New Injury, Initial Rehabilitation, Paraplegic

Partially compensatory system until mobility techniques are mastered
Goals:

1. Independent on discharge with continued educative-supportive nursing system on an episodic basis to aid adjustment
2. Independence complete within 2 years

The Nursing System, With a Focus on Nursing Actions in Relation to Levels of Nursing Agency

Professional

Accountable and responsible for the whole of the nursing system. Emphasis in practice: manages a caseload of complex nursing cases; identifies covert nursing problems; uses specialized nursing technologies as needed; discovers and validates new or improved technologies to solve nursing problems; skillfully uses social and interpersonal technologies, especially in working with groups of patients, families, and nursing personnel; develops authoritative and scholarly nursing documentation, verbal and written presentations; designs and develops nursing systems and establishes nursing standards for a specific patient population; oversees all patients on a disability category service—inpatients and outpatients—if assigned to a service or may provide specialty consultation, such as mental health.

Focus is on:

A. Self-care agency:

Promotion of capabilities: Unless acutely ill from complications, will cognitively be able to attend to, participate in, and practice therapeutic measures within physical limitations, can learn to perform new or adjusted self-care measures.

Self-care limitations:

1. Lack of awareness of alterations in body functioning: lack of mobility to monitor and regulate health condition and treatment related to spinal cord injury.

2. Lack of knowledge and skill to adjust prior self-care practices to altered condition and integrate into a daily therapeutic regime.

3. Variable ability to adjust to and accept disability and alterations in body and self-image.

4. Degree of motivation to learn and exercise self-care varies with sociocultural values, family support systems, personality, and life orientation of individual; some have no perception of need or willingness to acquire self-care knowledge and skills.

5. Variations in ability to control behavior to the extent needed for self-care and/or for permitting others to perform care and consistently tolerating constraints of rehabilitation regimen and adjusting to need for and services of dependent care agent (for some quadriplegics).

6. Extent of development of previous self-care system varies depending on age, values, interests, sociocultural orientation, and past life experiences as affected by the spinal cord injury.

Adolescents: Self-care agency is developing, may not be operative; inadequate to partially adequate.

Adults: Self-care agency is developed, not operative to partially operative; inadequate to partially adequate.

7. Ability to integrate self-care/dependent care with other aspects of daily living: initially may be inadequate.

8. Dependent care agent limitations: lack of knowledge and skill, willingness, and/or ability to assume the added responsibility and work required to assist another with self-care on a continuing daily basis for life; some lack the physical strength and stamina for this, especially older persons. Frequently, there is despair and resentment about maintaining the dependent at home or returning home on a permanent basis.

B. Self-care requisites:
Learn to manage health deviation self-care to:

1. Seek and cooperate with medical, nursing, and other therapies and diagnostic measures; follow schedule and practice prescribed measures; assert self in dealing with caregivers; make choices and decisions in planning care.

2. Become informed about, seek, and use available health care services and resources of the rehabilitation center—chaplain, psychologist, social worker, vocational rehabilitation, etc.—to overcome obstacles to self-care and integrated functioning.

3. Adjust or learn to live with alterations in body functioning and body image as affected by changes in sensation, perception, proprioception, self-image, and self-esteem; manage stress associated with injury and demands of health care environment.

4. Determine and seek resources to overcome obstacles to self-care at home: financial, physical equipment, supplies, personal assistance, and alterations in home, such as ramps, door, and bath.

Adjust and manage universal and developmental self-care requisites as altered by spinal cord injury:

1. Make decisions and choices about schedule of activities; pace self to conserve energy, prevent fatigue, and optimize strength; participate in social activities and rest as needed.

2. Adjust/review previous self-care knowledge and practices in relation to new demands and self-care limitations.

3. Accept, cooperate with, and/or directly manage care by dependent care agent.

4. Continue normal development adjusted to disability in relation to sexuality, social roles, family life, educational/occupational, and personal aspirations and activities.

5. Acquire new living skills, problem-solve, and make adjustments and decisions about how to deal with living environment—to physically and socially negotiate in community.

C. Nursing actions:

1. Assist the individual to cooperate with or engage in the therapeutic regime and to perform self-care and follow through actions around the clock in accord with prescribed therapies and his or her capabilities.

2. Assist patients to ask questions, make decisions about care measures and scheduling of activities, and seek help when needed; the nurse provides the help requested as appropriate.

3. Teach patients to monitor self and manage self-care, and validate learning of new or revised self-care techniques with patient/family.

4. Help individuals learn strengths and weaknesses, practice social roles appropriate to age and sex; encourage reality testing by promoting effort to try new things—trips to cafeteria or activity room; going on pass out of the hospital to movies or games; trial home visits; participation in group counseling, etc.

5. Assist to regulate activities for rest, scheduling, and pacing; reward for success, and set limits on excesses.

6. Detect problems in managing behavior detrimental to self-care and/or therapeutic regimen (e.g., inappropriate pain

management, excess anger, apathy, manipulative behavior, prolonged denial, hallucinations), and refer for appropriate mental health assistance and support in management.

7. Coordinate nursing with other therapies prescribed, and counsel and guide patients to seek and use the appropriate health care services.

8. Evaluate home situation for living accommodations requiring modification, equipment, results of trial home visits, and need for home health referral; in special situation, evaluate work and school environment.

9. Identify and work with family members/significant others as dependent care agents to learn self-care program and integrate it into system of daily living.

10. Provide information and counsel about seeking and using available health care resources, including financial, physical, and social resources, to overcome obstacles to self/dependent care; coordinate nursing actions with self-care procedures of patients taught by other therapists.

11. Provide follow-up evaluation, guidance and teaching, and support to patients as outpatients in clinic, on telephone, and on home visits.

Positions: Clinical nurse specialists (education level MSN) and rehabilitation nurse clinician (education level BSN with experience or certified rehabilitation RN). Work flexible time and place to meet patient needs (i.e., inpatient service, outpatient clinic, home).

Technical

Accountable and responsible for managing less complex nursing cases on the inpatient service or outpatient clinic; follows selected cases from admission through discharge from the hospital; serves as a team leader for an assigned group of patients and personnel. Emphasis in practice: identifies more common nursing problems; skillfully uses standardized validated nursing technologies.

Focus is on:

A. Skillful use of valid technologies to diagnose and regulate:

1. Movement of body: Paraplegia—has upper extremity movement but lacks knowledge and skill to alter body positions and use mobility devices and is unable to manage lower body and elimination functions. Quadriplegia—lower extremities immobile, and ability to move upper extremities, breathe, swallow, cough, talk, and move depends on level and severity of cervical cord injury. Improvement in time for either paraplegics or quadriplegics depends on whether cord injury is complete or incomplete.

2. Lack of knowledge and skill to adjust prior self-care practices to altered condition and integrate into daily therapeutic regimen.

3. Inability to control and pace activity/rest schedule to prevent or reduce fatigue in relation to decreased energy level.

4. All of the self-care limitations of interest to the professional, as listed previously.

B. Self-care requisites—all of those listed for the professional plus the following:

1. Learn to manage health deviation self-care to:

    1.1. Become aware of and monitor effects and results of spinal cord injury and treatment on self and body functioning.

    1.2. Acquire new knowledge and skills needed to monitor, prevent, and manage disability, other existing or potential health problems, and medications and treatments required (e.g., dysreflexia, urinary tract infection, skin breakdown, pain, spine instability, bracing and splints of body parts, and use of equipment).

    1.3. On inpatient admission, learn physical environment, routines, rules, and regulations of residence and operation of health care system as different from acute care institution; adjust to living with other patients and staff for extended period of time

2. Adjust and manage universal and developmental self-care requisites as altered by spinal cord injury:

   2.1. Monitor self in terms of new norms in body function and effectiveness of self-care measures to manage:

      2.1.1. Breathing, coughing, use of respirators and ventilation devices

      2.1.2. Elimination—bowel and bladder and complications, bathing

      2.1.3. Nutrition and hydration; eating techniques

      2.1.4. Mobility measures; prevention of pressure sores, contractures, and heterotopic ossification; control of spasticity; performance of range-of-motion exercises

      2.1.5. Infection—to prevent, detect, and treat pulmonary, genitourinary, skin infections

      2.1.6. Prevention of hazards—fractures, burns, skin trauma

      2.1.7. Temperature regulation—clothing and protective measures

   2.2. Manage regimen to control above and engage in activities of daily living using special assistive equipment—wheelchair, commode chair, etc.

   2.3. Develop and/or adjust self-care system to be compatible with lifestyle and family system in daily living.

C. Nursing actions:

1. Inform about hospital routines, rules, and procedures, what individual and family can expect from hospitalization and what they can or cannot do, who is available to help who is in charge and how to get help; orient to personnel and physical environment.

2. Monitor health statistics changes over time with respect to effects and results on integrated functioning from therapies, spinal cord injury, complications, etc. Assess physical, psychological adjustment, basic capabilities and disposition (e.g., cardiopulmonary changes, orthostatic hypotension, spinal shock, autonomic dysreflexia, thrombophlebitis, spasticity).

3. Institute and carry out prescribed medical and nursing measures to manage administration of medications, intravenous, assist with diagnostic and treatment procedures as needed on a continuing basis.

4. Assess self-care practices altered by disability and effects of disability on normal body functioning; monitor and regulate respiration, etc.

5. Assist the individual to cooperate with or engage in the therapeutic regime and to perform self-care, and follow through actions around the clock in accord with prescribed therapies and his or her capabilities.

6. Assist patients to ask questions, make decisions about care measures and scheduling of activities, and seek help when needed; the nurse provides the help requested as appropriate.

7. Teach patients to monitor self and manage self-care, and validate learning of new or revised self-care techniques with patient/family.

8. Help individuals learn strengths and weaknesses, practice social roles appropriate to age and sex; encourage reality testing by promoting effort to try new things—trips to cafeteria or activity room, going on pass out of hospital to movies or games, trial home visits, participation in group counseling, etc.

Positions: Rehabilitation nurse (advanced clinical RN position); general staff nurse (education level AD, BSN, diploma). Work assigned by place and shift.

Vocational

Responsible for skilled performance of assigned routine nursing tasks under supervision of a registered nurse. Emphasis in practice: Carries out routine assignment skillfully using standardized techniques in implementation of less complex care.

Positions: Licensed vocational/practical nurse, nursing assistant (education level, 1 year of formal education to 6- to 8-week training program for assistants).

Program Design in a Community Setting

T he following are excerpts from "Philosophy of Community Health Nursing":

> Nursing provides services within a multicultural community to people at all stages of development and in all health states. The particular service that nursing provides is an assisting one. That assistance can be offered through episodic or continual contact. What is accomplished directly or indirectly through nursing is an enhanced capacity for self-care by individuals, families and communities of persons so that they can achieve and maintain optimal health.

> Assistance offered by community health nurses is based on the belief that:
> 1. Requirements for self-care are common to all human beings and are learned within the context of social groups by communication and human interaction.

AUTHORS' NOTE: The forms and extracts in this appendix come from unpublished documents of the Vancouver Health Department, Vancouver, Canada. Materials reprinted courtesy of the Vancouver/Richmond Health Board.

2. Some requirements for self-care result from illness related limitations, which make self-care difficult or impossible.
3. Self-care actions are deliberate actions learned and performed to meet and know needs for care.
4. People's beliefs and values about health and self-care actions are inseparably linked to ethnic and cultural customs.

The following is an excerpt from "Standards for Nursing Practice":

The major focus of nursing is the promotion of health related self-care. This is accomplished by working with individuals, families, and community groups.

The following is an excerpt from "Assessment Standards":

Actions to Be Taken by Child (Self-Care Demand)	Knowledge, Skill, Ability of Child to Take Action (Self-Care Agency)	Action to Be Taken by Caregiver in Relation to Child (Dependent Care Demand)	Knowledge, Skill, Ability to Take Action (Dependent Care Agency)
Maintaining a Balance Between Solitude and Social Interaction			
Provides cues about need for solitude/social interaction	Provides cues for solitude and social interaction	Responds to cues appropriately	Is able to interpret cues; is aware of own and child's need for social contact
Plays by self Socializes appropriately with peers, adults	Is able to attend, initiate play by self Is willing to try new social experiences	Provides appropriate activities to encourage play Provides positive conditions for socializing	Knows about play as learning, play materials

Actions to Be Taken by Child (Self-Care Demand)	Knowledge, Skill, Ability of Child to Take Action (Self-Care Agency)	Action to Be Taken by Caregiver in Relation to Child (Dependent Care Demand)	Knowledge, Skill, Ability to Take Action (Dependent Care Agency)
		Promotion of Language Development	
Increasing understanding of what is being said	Is able to attend, hear, listen Retrieves the right words to express thoughts	Monitors for signs of hearing; seeks appropriate help if not present	Knows techniques for checking hearing (e.g., child's responses to name, localizing sound)
Is aware of self as individual	Gives first and last name	Uses child's correct name in positive manner	
		Respects/is aware of child as individual progressing toward independence	
Is able to accurately name objects, relate experience	Verbally relates own experience to action/ideas		
Is able to learn, remember new words		Provides opportunities, listens, role-models, integrates language with everyday activities	Understands how children learn
		Provides daily opportunities to encourage use of words; introduces and repeats new words in context	
		Is willing to take time; knows about age-appropriate books and experiences to promote language	

The Clinical
Communication System

As in any large-scale human service organization, formal and informal communication within the health care enterprise is a key to production of quality services. It is key to achieving the goals and maintaining the integrity of the enterprise, to interdisciplinary activity and relationships, to quality control mechanisms, and to research and development. The purpose of the communication system is not only to share information across the system but to assemble useful pertinent data in a usable form. The focus in this chapter is on the part that the clinical information system plays or can play in facilitating the design and production of the nursing component of patient/client care and the utility of nursing theory in constructing the clinical information system.

Developing a System to Document the
Nursing Component of Patient Care

Nurses, as well as others in health care, frequently are resistant to doing "more paperwork." Many feel they have more than they can contend with now without being required to do more writing. A study by Tapp (1990) listed inhibitors to documentation, such as lack of time, space, and language. A theoretical framework is cited as one of the facilitators to nursing documentation; thus, structuring of such forms from a theoretical perspective, as discussed in this chapter, may contribute to minimizing nurses' time and effort. Standardization of documentation forms and tools and computerization of information are all means to facilitate documentation, but the system chosen must not be burdensome. If nursing is to be more than procedures and routines, then deliberative effort must be given to documentation—the content, forms, and technologies—when designing and developing nursing systems. When the documentation reflects the concerns of nursing practice, and when nurses see it as meaningful to patient care beyond meeting accreditation requirements or institutional standards, the resistance to documentation is lessened. Use of the self-care deficit nursing theory to guide the construction of documentation tools can facilitate the documentation process and identification of nursing outcomes.

Issues in Developing a Documentation System

Each institution or agency usually develops its own forms and tools for nursing assessments and documentation of patient progress. The main problem is to keep them salient to each patient situation, to reduce redundancy (not copy information readily available elsewhere in the record), and to make the information meaningful to any nurse or other health care provider who picks up and reads the patient's record. Sometimes there is a tendency to collect too much information, to "cover all bases" in case of need. Some institutions document by exception: That is, all is considered satisfactory or not relevant unless recorded. Often, too, excellent assessments are done without documentation or follow-up of findings in terms of change or maintenance in self-care and self-care capabilities in progress notes or a nursing discharge summary.

With today's pressures for economy and compliance with documentation requirements necessary for reimbursement purposes, the nurse must learn to home in on what is most important as quickly and thoroughly as possible. When a theory such as the self-care deficit nursing theory is used to guide the data collection process, the nurse has some structure for interviewing patients and collecting data. Structured instruments for data gathering are helpful but should not limit the nurse. All of his or her other knowledge and skills based on experience are needed to readily (even intuitively) identify what needs to be done and when or why, with estimation of anticipated results. Recording systems, manual or computerized, must not only facilitate initial assessments but promote easy updating of progress and revision of nursing prescriptions and goals. The data collected and plans made must be meaningful to other nurses who share in the care process and to other members of the health care team.

Some years ago, nursing data collection forms and methods for assessment in a nurse-conducted clinic for diabetic patients were designed so that the patient and/or unlicensed nursing personnel could gather much of the data. The registered nurse then reviewed it to further explore areas of relevance. The nurse practitioner in this clinic commented that it took longer to do a thorough nursing assessment than to do a medical one because she had to know all that the patient knew and was doing in order for them to develop a realistic daily plan of care together. Over the years, many different tools and forms derived from self-care deficit nursing theory have been developed to meet the needs of particular institutions and patient populations. Some have been published; most have not.

The Importance of Staff Involvement

Involving staff in the development of data collection tools is absolutely necessary. They are the end users and must find the tools useful and meaningful. They also have practical knowledge about what information is important, how to collect it, and how to record it. When an institution is introducing the requirement to collect data about new variables, as in the case of introducing the self-care perspective, staff can learn, through participation in tool development, about the dimensions and attributes of the new variables. Staff may also require education programs for greater understanding of the variables of concern. Experience has demonstrated that staff frequently have difficulty identifying the indicators of capabilities necessary for self-care: for example, indicators that a person has the knowledge on which to base a decision about a particular self-care practice. Also, they know the nursing role in relation to meeting the self-care requisites but have difficulty describing the data indicating that a particular self-care requisite is or is not being met. Staff are used to collecting data and recording information about basic conditioning factors such as medical diagnosis and treatment plan. They are not used to using that information specifically in reference to the impact of these factors on the self-care system and recording information about that impact. This is the missing piece in many of the current records that purport to document nursing.

Nursing Forms

In most health care organizations, forms are used to document nursing, even though nursing data can easily be recorded on a blank sheet of paper. Forms facilitate recording of relevant information and ensure some consistency in data collection. Examples of forms for use in rehabilitation, community health, and acute care settings based on self-care deficit nursing theory can be found in Appendices 7A, 7B, and 7C. Note that these forms use the same categories of data as were identified in Chapter 4's Appendix 4A as being useful for describing patient populations. These forms summarize data for nursing care planning and documentation of patient progress from admission through discharge. The first set of forms is designed for a rehabilitation inpatient population, and the second set is for clients in community settings. The categories of data and many of the items on the forms are applicable to any nursing population. The forms are constructed to be applicable to computerization and to identify nursing outcomes (discussed in Chapter 8). The forms have been developed by staff nurses who were experts in their field, with input from persons familiar with nursing theory to help provide a systematic format for structuring the forms.

Using Nursing Theory to Specify Elements of a Computer-Based Clinical Nursing Information System and an Information-Processing Model

Bliss-Holtz and colleagues (Bliss-Holtz, McLaughlin, & Taylor, 1990; Bliss-Holtz, Taylor, & McLaughlin, 1992; Bliss-Holtz, Taylor, McLaughlin, Sayers, & Nickle, 1992; McLaughlin, Taylor, Bliss-Holtz, Sayers, & Nickle, 1990) specified the elements of a computer-based clinical nursing information system and an information-processing model derived from self-care deficit nursing theory—the result of a cooperative effort involving nursing theorists, practitioners of nursing, nursing researchers, and computer specialists. The practitioners of nursing described the information required in their day-to-day practice and how it was used. The theorists analyzed the information and the information-processing operations described by the practitioners. From this, they used nursing theory to develop a nursing process model and then an information-processing model. The researchers validated the models in practice settings. The computer specialists developed the computer prototype.

   Nursing theory provided direction for developing the data entry structure and processes, the data dictionary, and the logic for information management. As a result, a large number of data elements were made available for manipulation, resulting in the ability to produce reports for a variety of purposes, including patient management, research, program planning, and financial decision making. These data elements reflected the variables of concern in the provision of nursing services: the basic conditioning factors, including personal sociocultural factors, health state and health care system, family system, conditions and patterns of living, and developmental factors; the actions required to meet self-care requisites; and the capabilities of patients/clients to take the required action. For example:

1. The data element of "blood pressure of 200/110 mm Hg" is entered into a record that also includes information that the patient is a 66-year-old man who is homeless.

2. These data elements are linked to the components of the self-care system most likely to be affected by these conditioning factors, including maintaining a sufficient intake of food, maintaining a balance between rest and activity, promoting normalcy, seeking and securing medical assistance, monitoring health state, carrying out prescribed diagnostic and therapeutic measures, and learning to live with the effects of a particular pathological state.

3. Information is entered into the system that indicates the inability of the client/patient to adjust the self-care actions as required to manage this elevated blood pressure in terms of factors associated with knowledge, decision making, and production of self-care and with foundational capabilities and dispositions and their conditioning effects.

4. From the above data, a plan of action can be generated.

5. The results of the plan of action can be tracked at specific points in time.

6. Patient records with similar data elements can be compared and contrasted to
   - Develop critical path and case management guidelines
   - Evaluate outcomes of nursing interventions
   - Link patient outcomes with characteristics of staff providing service
   - Determine the particular characteristics of the patient population being served
   - Develop care and prevention programs specific to the patient subpopulation
   - Specify costs of service provided to particular patient subpopulations

Samples of data entry and output for a population during the first 48 hours postpartum are included in Tables 7.1 and 7.2.

The Importance of the Clinical Information System

For purposes of this chapter, clinical information is any information pertaining to individual clients/patients and or groups of patients that is directly concerned

TABLE 7.1 Sample of Data Input for Computer Information System

Data items are for a patient in the first 48 hours postpartum.

The components of the therapeutic self-care demand are listed. Beside each, the nurse will indicate limitations in meeting this requisite by indicating if the limitation is related to knowing (K), decision making (D), acting (A), or a combination, such as DA, decision making and acting. For example:

Limitations in maintaining a balance between rest and activity:

K	Adjusting to baby's asleep/awake pattern
A	Adjusting to sleeping in a strange environment
A	Feeding baby in restful position
	Soliciting help to care for baby
K	Prioritizing energy expenditure
DA	Incorporating postpartum exercises into exercise schedule
A	Practicing good body mechanics

with delivery of patient care. It includes the information documented in the patient/client record, standards of care, protocols and procedures related to provision of care, and specified outcomes. The clinical information system includes the written documents associated with the components and the formal and informal verbal exchanges that take place between caregivers.

TABLE 7.2 Sample of Output From Computer Information System Based on Input From Table 7.1

In addition to generating individual care plans based on the input, the following kinds of reports can be generated in relation to the population:

Patients on the unit lacking knowledge concerning infant/sleep awake patterns:

Room 108a	Jane Brown
Room 115	Susan Jones
Room 105b	Mary Smith

or:

Patients on the unit needing assistance with exercise program:

Room 118	June Good
Room 105	Mary Smith
Room 112	Sally Green

Year-end summary data could include the number of patients who at 12 hours, 24 hours, and 48 hours were not able to meet specific self-care requisites. This information would assist in program planning for early discharges from the unit.

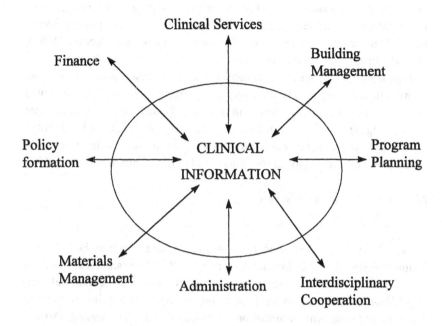

Figure 7.1. Importance of Clinical Information System

The health care industry has been interested in development of patient/ clinical information systems for over 30 years. However, although banks spend about 12% of their operating budgets on information systems, only 2% is spent by businesses that are providers of health care (Renner & Swart, 1997). Patient/ client data are central to any health care enterprise information system. The importance of the clinical information system to the operation of the health care enterprise is illustrated in Figure 7.1. The information about the patients and their care is used for the care process, reimbursement, quality improvement, statistical reporting, health care planning, education, research, and litigation (Nelson, 1997). Organizing, manipulating, controlling, and presenting these data are essential processes related to productivity and to decision making.

Clinical Information and
Management for Nursing Purposes

Persons responsible for the delivery of nursing services require information to support and inform management of individual patient care, management of patient care units, management of groups of patients, program planning, design of the patient/nursing services, management of those services, resource allocation and utilization, personnel management, and policy making. Simpson (1996), claiming that "information is power," stated, "The effective practice of nursing is dependent on the ability of clinical nurses and nurse managers to locate relevant information quickly and interpret it correctly" (p. 86). However, much of the information that is pertinent to the practice of nursing and the management of a nursing service either has not been recorded or is embedded in handwritten records in a format that makes it unretrievable, or retrievable only if expensive "hand searches" are employed (and thus for all practical purposes inaccessible).

Management of Data by Nurses
for Non-Nursing Purposes

Nurses manage information not only for nursing purposes but also for virtually every other function and department within the health care enterprise as they process orders, requisition services, report results, initiate financial data, requisition supplies, and so on. In addition, much of nursing time is spent in handling and processing information for purposes other than nursing. Despite this, nurses seldom have access to modern information and electronic transfer communication systems that have been designed to serve their needs (Hannah & Anderson, 1994).

Issues in Electronic Processing of Clinical Data

Most clinical databases that are easily accessed electronically include demographic information, medical diagnoses and associated treatments in the form of surgical procedures and medications prescribed, length of stay/service delivery, and physician billing data. Superimposed on these data may be supplies used and staffing costs over particular time periods. Access to such information electronically is possible because these variables are easily identified and quantified. Computer-based admission, transfer, and discharge programs containing much of this information are in place in most health care enterprises, as are computer-based inventory programs, laboratory order/reporting systems, and physician order entry systems. However, much clinical information important to the health care planning and service delivery processes either is not collected systematically or is not available for analysis because of the recording and documentation system in place. For clinical information to be useful in the service delivery planning process, it must be collected systematically and recorded in such a way that it can be easily extracted and manipulated. Collecting data systematically involves identifying the variables of concern and the data in relation to those variables that are significant. The use of electronic databases for extraction and manipulation of the data should be a standard in today's world. However, before the data can be extracted, it must be entered into the system in a meaningful fashion. Nursing administration has a responsibility to develop and implement documentation systems from which the data necessary for designing and delivering nursing for populations cost-effectively can be retrieved. This begins with ensuring that the variables of concern to nursing are included in the system.

Traditionally, nursing documentation simply records procedures done, such as personal hygiene activities; medical orders carried out, such as medications and treatments given; observations made of the patient; and, perhaps, some teaching given, particularly in relation to medications. The essence of nursing too long has gone unrecognized and remained invisible because patient records reveal so little about actual nursing goals and results in terms of what the patient knows, does, and can do in managing his or her own health care and how the nurse deals with this. When nursing theory helps make the nursing contribution clear, nursing becomes visible in the patient's record. Moreover, definitive information about nursing can aid in the identification of nursing costs for administrative purposes.

Gabriell (1997) proposed that clinical thinking shift from evaluating patient status at a particular point in time, a snapshot perspective, to thinking of patient characteristics over time, a temporal perspective that allows for consideration of current data with past data. However, such a perspective is almost impossible with the current cumbersome written patient record and is even more impossible from a nursing perspective because the data required to obtain this perspective in relation to the concerns of nursing identified in Appendices 4A and 7A are frequently missing from the record.

The Clinical Information System and Operationalizing the Mission Statement and Goals

As described in Chapter 5, the mission statement sets forth the beliefs and purposes for the existence of an organization and provides direction for goal development. Clinical practice should be consistent with and concerned with achieving the stated goals. In turn, the clinical information system should reflect and be consistent with the mission statement and goals. The particular information that health care professionals are directed to complete as part of the patient record or data that must be gathered in compliance with procedures, protocols, and prescribed standards or achievement of identified outcomes all provides direction for and to a greater or lesser extent controls practice. If these structural components are not consistent with the mission statement and goals, it cannot be expected that clinical practice will be consistent with them. This consistency is illustrated in Appendix 7B.

The Clinical Information System and the Mental Model of Nursing

Major documentation of nursing concerns in many institutions has been located in nurses' notes, care plans, and cardex systems of some sort. In many cases, these have not formed part of the permanent record. The information contained in them has not formed part of the discharge summary, nor has it been incorporated into management reports of any sort. Hence, there is no permanent record of the bulk of the concern of nursing and nursing activity and no way to incorporate this information into program planning and resource allocation decisions.

The content of the clinical information system provides a perspective on what nursing is and what nurses do, and it communicates a certain perspective to all who have access to that information. When the information that can be readily accessed is primarily a reporting of observations relating to physiological status, treatments performed, and medications administered, that becomes the view of what nursing is all about. Heartfield (1996) suggested that the influence of ethical, legal, medical, and institutional guidelines has resulted in a "sanitation" such that what is recorded barely represents what has actually been done for the person. Heartfield pointed out that nurses often are dealing with intimate events that people do not want to know about. Also, nursing documentation is primarily in relation to the performance of medical orders and patient responses. Heartfield found that nurses write about observations and responses in a passive manner, providing a record of information that assists other health care providers but is devoid of meaning about nursing. The knowledge base underlying nursing activity is not apparent. Although the recordings of other health care workers include their judgments and examinations, nurses' recordings do not. Nurses also appear to value oral communication, much of which is nurse to nurse and is not available to the clinical information system at large (Parker & Gardner, 1992). Thus, nursing becomes the invisible service.

TABLE 7.3 Sampling of Minimum Data Sets

Uniform Hospital Discharge Data Set (UHDDS; U.S. Department of Health and Human Services, 1985).

Financial Uniform Minimum Data Set (UB-92; Ohio Hospital Association, 1992).

Uniform Ambulatory Care Data Set (U.S. Department of Health and Human Services, 1981; Revised 1989 and 1994).

Minimum Data Set: Multistate Nursing Home Case Mix and Quality Demonstration (Minimum Data Set, 1992).

Data Elements for Emergency Department Systems (DEEDS) Version 1.0. (Division of Acute Care, 1996).

Nursing Minimum Data Set (Werley & Lang, 1988).

Health Information: Nursing Component (Canadian Nurses Association, 1993).

Korner Minimum Data Set (National Health Service, 1982).

Health Medical Records Institute (HMRI; HMRI, 1991).

Medicaid-Medicare Common Data Initiative (Health Care Financing Administration, 1994).

Community Nursing Minimum Data Set (Gliddon & Weaver, 1994).

Nursing Minimum Data Set (Sermeus & Delesie, 1994).

The Importance of Language in the Clinical Information System

---

As identified by McCormick, Renner, Mayes, Regan, and Greenberg (1997), more than 17 minimum data sets have been developed in the health care field in the United States. Canada and countries in Europe have also developed such data sets. These include data sets developed to reflect services provided in hospitals, long-term care, community, emergency, ambulatory care, home care, and hospice settings, as well as services for financial purposes and professional services. A sample list of the data sets is shown in Table 7.3.

A comparison of the data elements included demonstrates that the data sets have some commonality. However, data that inform the practice of nursing and delivery of nursing services are still incomplete. The contribution that a nursing practice theory can make to the development of such data sets is illustrated in Table 7.4. A sampling of data sets, data included in those sets, and variables of concern to nursing as identified by self-care deficit nursing theory are presented. The items proposed include data elements of interest to the nurse in each patient/client encounter and can be included in the documentation system. Including them in the documentation system facilitates extraction of these elements in preparing current and historical reports for administrative purposes. Discharge summaries can inform national research and planning bodies.

TABLE 7.4 Data Items: Minimum Data Sets and Self-Care Deficit Nursing Theory

UHDDS	Korner MDS	HMRI	NMDS	HI:NC	SCDNT
		Demographics and Care Items			
Client ID	Date of birth	Health care no.	Client ID	Unique lifetime ID	Lifetime ID
Date of birth	Sex	Date of birth/age	Date of birth		Date of birth/age
Sex		Sex	Sex		Sex
Medical diagnosis	Medical diagnosis	Medical diagnosis (primary, secondary)	Nursing diagnosis	Client status	Adequacy of self-care/dependent care management system
Procedure and dates	Operative procedure		Nursing intervention	Nursing intervention	
			Intensity of nursing care	Nursing intensity	Nursing system/intensity
			Nursing outcome	Cliet outcomes	
					Health care system factors
					Medical diagnosis/treatments, studies, other therapies
Race, ethnicity			Race, ethnicity	Language	Personal/sociocultural, including education level, literacy, language(s), and occupation
				Occupation	
				Education level	
				Literacy level	
				Income level	Available resources
					Family system factors
					Developmental care system

Residence	Residence	Postal code	Residence	Living arrangements	Conditions of living
				Home environment	Patterns of living
				Work environment	
				Functional health status	Self-care system, self-care deficit
				Lifestyle data	
				Caregiver on discharge	Dependent care unit, dependent care deficit, dependent care system
				Burden on caregiver	

Service Items

Facility/agency no.	Health district no.	Provider/institution no.	Facility/agency no.	Unique nurse ID	Unique nurse ID
Attending physician ID	Code of GP or consultant	Chart no.	Health record no.	Principal nurse provider	Nurse provider(s)
Operating MD	Right of admission	Responsible MD	Principal nurse ID		Admission date
Admission date	Nursing episode code	Responsible consultant	Disposition of patient		Discharge date
Discharge date	Admission date	Admission date/hour			Disposition
Disposition of patient	Admission source	Institution from			
	Admission method	Admission category			
	Consult	Ambulance			
	Length of stay	Live/death codes			
	Nursing home	Length of stay			
	Operational plan	Discharge date/hour			
	Destination of discharge/transfer	Responsibility for payment			
	Method of discharge	Main patient service			
	Category of patient				

NOTE: UHDDS, Uniform Hospital Discharge Data Set (U.S. Department of Health and Human Services, 1985); Korner MDS, Korner Minimum Data Set (National Health Service, 1982); HMRI, Health Medical Records Institute Minimum Data Set (HMRI, 1991); NMDS, Nursing Minimum Data Set (Werley & Lang, 1988); HI:NC, Health Information, Nursing Component (Canadian Nurses Association, 1993); SCDNT, self-care deficit nursing theory.

For many years, the language of nursing and the language of medicine appeared to be synonymous. This implied that the variables of concern to medicine and nursing were the same, and the variables identified in the patient record about which information was gathered frequently reflected this belief. With the identification of the proper object of nursing and the development of nursing theories that specify the focus of nursing, it has become evident that nursing is concerned not only with the variables of concern to medicine but also with other variables, as illustrated in Appendix 4A and Chapter 2. It has also become evident that the goals of medicine and nursing, though related and interdependent, are not the same. These developments have made it clear that nursing needs a language of its own to describe its focus of concern—a language that can be the basis for the development of an information system reflective of nursing concerns.

Lang (1995), a prime mover in the development of the nursing minimum data set, stated that nurses need to have a language beyond medical language to talk about nursing. She suggested that rather than talking about what nurses do for patients with, for example, a hip fracture, such a conversation should include questions about what nurses do for patients' pain, confusion, mobility, incontinence, dehydration, and so on. It is our contention that it is important to talk about more than what nurses do for patients and that self-care deficit nursing theory provides the means for doing this.

The items of concern that Lang suggested are consistent with and partially descriptive of nursing. They fall under the rubric of the basic conditioning factor of health state (the hip fracture, pain, confusion, mobility, incontinence, and dehydration). All of them influence the actions to be taken to meet the self-care requisites and the capability of individuals to take the required action. In other words, they influence the self-management system that is appropriate to the situation. Rather than talking about what nurses "do" for persons having had a hip fracture who have pain, confusion, mobility, incontinence, and so on, the focus of concern becomes, "How does a fractured hip affect the self-care system?"—that is, "What different care measures are required to meet the self-care requisites, which capabilities are required now and which in the future, and does the patient have those capabilities?" Subsequent to that, the concern is, "What nursing care is required at this point in time and over time to enable the person to meet his or her self-care requisites now and in the future?" Thus, self-care deficit nursing theory not only supports Lang's contention that these are areas of concern to nursing but provides direction to nurses to act proactively rather than reactively. It provides nurses with a way of thinking about the patient situation, thus freeing them from merely following rules and protocols. It facilitates thinking about the patient situation in a holistic fashion and provides direction for collecting data, for anticipating and identifying problems, and for determining appropriate actions.

The language of nursing must also provide names for and a way of describing the whole of nursing. Although described elsewhere, these are repeated here for review purposes: the nature of the entities of concern, the processes of nursing, and the patterns of behavior. From observation, study, and analysis of nursing practice situations, nursing is concerned with persons who are unable, for health-related reasons, to meet their continuous requirements for self-care (Orem, 1995, 1997). Meeting their continuous requirements for self-care includes knowing these requirements and acting to meet them. The actions that are required have been named the *therapeutic self-care demand*. Nursing is concerned with persons who are unable to meet the health-related self-care requirements of dependents (*dependent care demand*). Nursing is concerned with the three human powers: self-care agency, dependent care agency, and nursing agency. *Self-care agency* is the power to develop and exercise capabilities to know and meet the therapeutic self-care demand. *Dependent care agency* is the power to develop and exercise capabilities to know the dependent care demand so as to ensure that the therapeutic self-care demand of the socially dependent person is met. *Nursing agency* is the power to design and produce nursing care for others. Conditioning factors influence therapeutic self-care demand, dependent care demand, self-care agency, dependent care agency, and nursing agency.

Therefore, nurse managers and administrators of nursing services concerned with productivity and decision making relating to design and delivery of nursing must have information systems that facilitate the collection and manipulation of data about the conditioning factors, therapeutic self-care demand, dependent care demand, self-care agency, and dependent care agency of persons making up the population served (see Appendix 4A). A detailed description of these variables and their relationships is provided in Chapter 2. Data pertinent to these variables must be included in discharge planning summaries from which information is abstracted for national databases used in health care planning.

The Clinical Information System: An Integral Component of the Management Information System

Administrators of nursing services have available to them automated reporting systems that generate reports about salary and supply budgets, workload measurement, resource utilization, quality management, patient/client demographics, and so on. Shamian and Hannah (1995) suggested that these information systems lack indicators about the level, quality, appropriateness, cost, and clinical outcomes of care delivered to a specific patient. It is frequently not possible to relate ambulatory care to inpatient information. The materials are presented in a linear fashion representing only a point in time, and identifying best practices is almost impossible because of a lack of standardization of indicators and terminology. Also, because of the lack of time between episodes of care and processing of the information, the data are often outdated. The authors concluded that "overall, nurse executives are left to cope with management information systems that are data rich and information poor" (p. 204).

At the heart of the problem with many of the automated information systems available is the source data for those systems. As indicated previously, reports are compiled from data more appropriate to finances, materials management, admission-transfer-discharge, laboratory functioning, and pharmacy operation than to management of services associated with nursing and are not complete for purposes of nursing administration. The clinical data are composed of records of treatments, medications, and tests performed, which are reflective of medical activity but again are inadequate for nursing purposes. The patient variables of therapeutic self-care demand, the characteristics of self-care agency, the conditioning factors affecting the patient situation, and the nature of their conditioning effect, which in turn influence the quantity and quality of nursing services required, are not addressed. In addition, nursing theory has not been used to inform the information-processing model; hence, it does not address the relationships of the variables of concern to nursing.

Information management will continue to be an ongoing issue for nursing administration. Efforts and research projects to facilitate nursing management decisions include the following significant projects:

- The development of the client record and information management system by the Visiting Nurse Association of Omaha, Nebraska
- The formation of the North American Nursing Diagnosis Association (NANDA)
- The impetus of Werley in the development of the minimum data set
- The development of the Iowa Nursing Interventions Classification
- The development of the Georgetown Intervention Classification
- The development of the Iowa Nursing Outcome Classification

Each of these developments is a significant step in the task of trying to manage data related to the practice of nursing. A significant omission to date has been the lack of such developments from the perspective of the nursing theories. Taylor (1990) initiated discussion about a taxonomy related to nursing diagnosis. Bliss-Holtz (1996) described initial efforts at generating diagnostic statements for electronic documentation.

The Nursing Management Minimum Data Set

Huber, Schumacher, and Delaney (1997) expressed a need for a nursing management minimum data set that would enable nurse executives to identify the effectiveness of nursing within the broader health care system. They described 17 elements of a nursing management minimum data set that have been developed through a consensus process involving nurse executives and nurse researchers. These elements have been placed in three categories: environment, nurse resources, and financial resources. As illustrated in the following discussion, development of indicators particularly related to those falling within the category of environment can be facilitated by use of self-care deficit nursing theory.

Huber et al. suggested that the nurse executive should be able to describe precisely the types of nursing unit/service, the patient/client population(s) served, the volume of nursing delivery by unit/service, the complexity of clinical decision making, and the complexity of the environment. As has been repeatedly demonstrated throughout this book, a nursing theory such as self-care deficit nursing theory specifies the variables and provides direction for development of a clinical information system that can provide the nurse executive with just such data. Without such a nursing theory, there is no basis for specifying the required information or the means of collecting it.

The nurse resources category includes nursing staff satisfaction and client satisfaction. For this information to have meaning for the nurse executive in responding to the tensions between budget and staffing needs, there must be a means of linking this information to patient variables of concern to nursing. The nursing theory provides direction for identifying the patient variables and for developing an information system whereby these data can be linked.

The financial resources category includes nursing delivery unit/service budget. Using nursing theory to specify patient variables and linking these to the nursing unit/service budget will enable nurse executives to precisely relate nursing service delivery, nursing outcomes, and expenditures. It should also enable nurse executives to estimate the relationship of activities of other professional persons to nursing costs. The clinical data that the nurse uses to manage the care of individuals and populations can and should be the basis for the nursing management data set. Nursing theory helps to specify those data.

The Clinical Information System and
Nursing Workload/Patient Classification Reporting

For more than 30 years, nurses have completed patient classification reports for the purpose of determining workload. Although these classification reports are based on clinical information that is frequently duplicated in the patient record, there are no systems in place that we know of that allow for electronic extraction of this information from the record. Basing the nursing component of the clinical information system and the patient classification system on the same theoretical system would allow for development of such a system.

Completion of the classification reports purportedly should have helped to predict and specify staffing requirements and resource allocation based on patient need. O'Brien-Pallas (1988) and O'Brien-Pallas, Leatt, Dever, and Till (1989) found that estimates of absolute hours of care provided by three commonly used systems (GRASP, PRN, and Medicus) differed significantly when all three tools were used on the same patient population. In surveying staff nurses, Cockerill and O'Brien-Pallas (1990a) found that the most common objection to the workload measurement system was that it did not reflect true workload. In addition, staff nurses stated that the staffing was not adjusted to the workload identified and that the measurement systems were too time consuming to complete. Cockerill and O'Brien-Pallas (1990b) also found that users of the systems wanted the following items included in future systems:

- Clinical judgment of the nurse
- Theoretical model for nursing
- Patient condition/nursing diagnosis
- Decision models
- Integration of standards of nursing practice and quality of care measures

Using self-care deficit nursing theory as a basis for nursing practice, including development of patient classification systems and workload measurement systems, facilitates incorporating these items into the clinical information system in a logical and theoretically consistent manner. When a nursing practice theory such as self-care deficit nursing theory is used to direct practice in an institution and to develop the nursing component of the clinical information system, the items that currently make up the patient classification systems, the nursing workload indexes, and the items identified above as part of the "wish" lists can be a by-product of the clinical information system.

The Clinical Information System and
the Health Care Planning Process

The importance of and lack of an adequate integrated database for health care planning have been identified in both Canada (Canadian Nurses Association, 1993) and the United States (Swart, 1997). There has been a great deal of interest in the development of a minimum data set for nursing (Canadian Nurses Association, 1993; Werley & Lang, 1988) and, more widely in the health care field, the development of a patient care minimum data set. McCormick et al. (1997) reported the identification of 17 minimum data sets developed in the United States by either the federal government or private enterprise. For the most part, the data sets in existence identify demographic information, dates or length of service, services utilized/provided, diagnostic tests performed, medical diagnoses, treatments, medications, review of body systems, past medical history, illness, and exposure to hazards.

In reviewing the databases, it would appear that data reflective of the interest of the medical profession, epidemiologists, and agencies funding health programs are included. Although this information has meaning to the development and delivery of nursing services, it is incomplete for purposes of determining the need for those services, designing them, managing delivery, and evaluating the service provided. Nursing data elements are absent from discharge abstracts of medical records departments in both Canada and the United States and are consequently absent from the national databases that are used for funding allocation and policy making (Hannah & Anderson, 1994). Hannah and Anderson reported, moreover, that these data elements also appear to be missing in European databases. This no doubt is partly because these data have not been included in the database input system and are difficult to retrieve from current clinical records. Nurses who do not work from a nursing-theory-based perspective have difficulty providing this information. It is incumbent on nursing administrators to work toward including data reflective of the need for nursing in these databases. Current work related to the development of the Nursing Intervention Classification and the Nursing Outcome Classification is an important contribution. However, much work remains to be done in relation to the nursing diagnosis component. This is work that cannot be done outside the clinical field and therefore requires leadership and cooperation from administrators of nursing services.

Summary

The importance of developing the nursing component of the clinical information system from a sound theoretical base has been described in this chapter. Such development contributes to informed management of the nursing service, informed health care planning, delivery of quality service, delivery of cost-effective service, nursing and patient care research, and development of nursing knowledge and the science of nursing. Development of such a system has not commonly occurred in the health care delivery system, where the needs of the medicine have been the primary organizer for the clinical communication system. Development of a clinical information system that also serves the needs of nursing is a challenge for the nurse administrator.

References

Bliss-Holtz, J. (1996). Using Orem's theory to generate nursing diagnoses for electronic documentation. *Nursing Science Quarterly, 9*(3), 121-125.

Bliss-Holtz, J., McLaughlin, K., & Taylor, S. (1990). Validating nursing theory for use within a computerized nursing information system. *Advances in Nursing Science, 13*(2), 46-52.

Bliss-Holtz, J., Taylor, S., & McLaughlin, K. (1992). Nursing theory as a base for a computerized nursing information system. *Nursing Science Quarterly, 5,* 124-128.

Bliss-Holtz, J., Taylor, S. G., McLaughlin, K., Sayers, P., & Nickle, L. (1992). Development of a computerized information system based on self-care deficit nursing theory. In J. Arnold & G. Pearson (Eds.), *Computer application in nursing education and practice* (pp. 87-93). New York: National League for Nursing.

Canadian Nurses Association. (1993). *Papers from the nursing minimum data set conference.* Ottawa: Author.

Cockerill, R. W., & O'Brien-Pallas, L. L. (1990a). Satisfaction with nursing workload systems: Report of a survey of Canadian hospitals, Part A. *Canadian Journal of Nursing Administration, 3*(3), 17-22.

Cockerill, R. W., & O'Brien-Pallas, L. L. (1990b). Satisfaction with nursing workload systems: Report of a survey of Canadian hospitals, Part B. *Canadian Journal of Nursing Administration, 3*(3), 23-26.

Division of Acute Care, Rehabilitation Research, and Disability Prevention, National Center for Injury Prevention and Control. (1996). *Data Elements for Emergency Department Systems (DEEDS), Version 1.0.* Atlanta, GA: Center for Disease Control and Prevention.

Gabriell, E. R. (1997). Longitudinal electronic patient records: A challenge of our time. *Computers in Nursing, 15*(2), S48-S52.

Gliddon, T., & Weaver, C. (1994). The community nursing minimum data set Australia: From definition to the real world. In S. J. Grobe & E. S. P. Pluyter-Wenting (Eds.), *Nursing informatics: An international overview for nursing in a technological era* (pp. 162-168). Amsterdam: Elsevier.

Hannah, K. J., & Anderson, B. J. (1994). Management of nursing information. In J. M. Hibberd & M. E. Kyle (Eds.), *Nursing management in Canada* (pp. 516-533). Toronto: W. B. Saunders.

Health Care Financing Administration, Office of Managed Care. (1994). *Medicaid-Medicare Common Data Initiative: A core data set for states and Medicaid managed care plans.*

Health Medical Records Institute. (1991). *HMRI abstracting manual.* Toronto: Author.

Heartfield, M. (1996). Nursing documentation and nursing practice: A discourse analysis. *Journal of Advanced Nursing, 24,* 98-103.

Huber, D., Schumacher, L., & Delaney, C. (1997). Nursing Management Minimum Data Set (NMMDS). *Journal of Nursing Administration, 27*(4), 43-48.

Lang, N. M. (1995). *Nursing data systems: The emerging framework.* Washington, DC: American Nurses Association.

McCormick, K., Renner, A. L., Mayes, R., Regan, J., & Greenberg, M. (1997). The federal and private sector roles in the development of minimum data sets and core health data elements. *Computers in Nursing, 15*(2, Suppl.), S23-S32.

McLaughlin, K., Taylor, S., Bliss-Holtz, J., Sayers, P., & Nickle, L. (1990). Shaping the future: The marriage of nursing theory and informatics. *Computers in Nursing, 8,* 174-179.

Minimum Data Set: Multistate nursing home case mix and quality demonstration training manual. (1992). Natick, MA: Eliot.

National Committee on Vital and Health Statistics. (1981). *Report of the National Committee on Vital and Health Statistics.* Hyattsville, MD: U.S. Department of Health and Human Services.

National Health Service (1982). *Korner Minimum Data Set.* London: Author.

Nelson, D. A. F. (1997). A defined minimum data set: Will it work for direct patient care? *Computers in Nursing, 15*(2, Suppl.), S43-S47.

O'Brien-Pallas, L. (1988). An analysis of multiple approaches to measuring nursing workload. *Canadian Journal of Nursing Administration, 1*(2), 8-11.

O'Brien-Pallas, L., Leatt, P., Dever, R., & Till, J. (1989). A comparison of workload estimates using three methods of patient classification. *Canadian Journal of Nursing Administration, 2*(3), 16-23.

Ohio Hospital Association. (1992). *Ohio Uniform Billing: 92 instructional manual.* Columbus, OH: Author.

Orem, D. E. (1995). *Nursing: Concepts of practice* (5th ed.). St. Louis, MO: C. V. Mosby.

Orem, D. E. (1997). Views of human beings specific to nursing. *Nursing Science Quarterly, 10*(1), 26-31.

Parker, J., & Gardner, G. (1992). The silence and the silencing of the nurse's voice: A reading of patient progress notes. *Australian Journal of Advanced Nursing, 9*(2), 3-9.

Renner, A., & Swart, J. C. (1997). Patient core data set: Standard for a longitudinal health/medical record. *Computers in Nursing, 15*(2), S7-S13.

Sermeus, W., & Delesie, L. (1994). The registration of a nursing minimum data set in Belgium: Six years of experience. In S. J. Grobe & E. S. P. Pluyter-Wenting (Eds.), *Nursing informatics: An international overview for nursing in a technological era* (pp. 144-149). Amsterdam: Elsevier.

Shamian, J., & Hannah, K. J. (1995). Management information systems for nurse executives. In M. J. Ball, K. J. Hannah, S. K. Newbold, & J. V. Douglas (Eds.), *Introduction to nursing informatics: Where caring and technology meet* (pp. 203-216). New York: Springer-Verlag.

Simpson, R. L. (1996). Information is power. *Nursing Administration Quarterly, 20*(3), 86-89.

Swart, J. C. (1997). A patient core data set and integrated health information system. *Computers in Nursing, 15*(2), 55-56.

Tapp, R. A. (1990). Inhibitors and facilitators to documentation in nursing practice. *Western Journal of Nursing Research, 12*, 229-240.

Taylor, S. T. (1990). The structure of nursing diagnoses from Orem's theory. *Nursing Science Quarterly, 4*(1), 24-32.

U.S. Department of Health and Human Services. (1985). 1984 revision of the Uniform Hospital Discharge Data Set. *Federal Register, 50*(147), 31-038 to 31-040.

Werley, H., & Lang, N. (Eds.). (1988). *Identification of the nursing minimum data set.* New York: Springer.

Nursing Documentation Forms
From a Rehabilitation Setting

Four nursing forms based on the problem-oriented approach to medical records are included in this appendix. The assessment form used for gathering data for the action plans and progress notes for the rehabilitation population is not included. The forms shown here summarize the assessment findings needed to determine the actions to be taken and indicate changes in self-care status that may occur. A variety of methods may be used to gather the information, such as physical inspection, interview, and consultation of other records. The forms shown present that information as conclusions drawn, judgments, and decisions made.

The first form, "Nursing Action Plan: Immediate," must be completed within 24 hours of admission. Note that this form provides for recording about patient capability in relation to specific requisites of concern:

- Establishing a communication system
- Controlling pain
- Managing processes related to bowel and bladder elimination
- Managing food and fluid intake
- Preventing hazards

AUTHORS' NOTE: The forms in this appendix were originally developed before 1990 in collaboration with the nurses at the Mississippi Methodist Rehabilitation Hospital and Center, Jackson, Mississippi. They are reprinted courtesy of the Nursing Department of the Mississippi Methodist Hospital and Rehabilitation Center.

Some specific patient/caregiver and nurse actions to meet the requisites are also addressed.

The second form, "Nursing Diagnosis: Admission/Discharge," lists potential nursing diagnoses. This form is used first on admission and again at the time of discharge. It provides for documenting specific information about self-care limitations and abilities in relation to identified requisites of concern for this patient population. Status relative to each diagnosis category listed and/or emergent categories can be evaluated for comparison at time of discharge to determine outcomes. This form also includes space for documentation about the caregivers (dependent care agents).

The third form, "Nursing Action Plan: Continuing," is designed to address areas that are not immediately discernible on admission and that the nurse has more time to investigate. This form is to be completed within the first week of hospitalization. It is used on a weekly basis from admission through discharge. It again addresses specified requisites of concern for this population and related actions.

The fourth form, "Self-Care Activities Flowsheet," lists the numerous activities to be managed by the patient, dependent care agent, and/or nursing personnel, and it provides for documentation of patient capability in relation to the specific activities.

The two action plan forms are based on the problem-oriented medical record system. Problems are numbered according to the order of priority. The layout seeks to identify the problems; the patient goals, with time anticipated for accomplishment, patient/caregiver actions; and nursing actions. To save writing time, many items can simply be checked by the nurse. Additional information can be written in on the form or on a separate blank nursing record sheet.

The approach on the immediate action form is to generally appraise the overall self-care system first (although in reality this may be done after evaluating the other items) and the reasons for the actions planned. The nursing diagnosis form more specifically addresses adequacy of actions—how well and how completely actions are performed—in terms of numbers of requisites met or unmet. The self-care requisites are predominantly those associated with spinal cord injury, brain injury, arthritis, and other disabling conditions. The particular developmental and health deviation self-care requisites are documented separately, although to some extent they are addressed on the continuing action plan and the flowsheet. There is also a space on the flowsheet to identify the status of the dependent care agent's abilities and actions.

NURSING ACTION PLAN: IMMEDIATE

(Complete on admission for next 24-48 hours
Number problems in order of priority)

# AND DATE PLUS SELF-CARE DEFICIT ACTUAL/ POTENTIAL (PROBLEM)	GOAL/TIME TO BE COMPLETED	PATIENT/ CAREGIVER ACTIONS	NURSING ACTIONS
USE OF KNOWLEDGE RE: ____ Call system ____ Hospital routines Associated with/related to:	Use nurse call as necessary, follow basic procedures	Document use of call system	Orient to: ____ Nurse call, unit routines, head nurse ____ Primary Nurse— visit min. 1 x per week ____ Bed operation, unit routines ____ Introduce roommate ____ Observe patient per routine ____ Other ____ Equipment within reach
TO COMMUNICATE RELATED TO:	Establish/use basic system to communicate	Help find a workable method	____ Locate room for observation ____ Develop alternative method ____ Eye blink ____ Gesture ____ Device ____ Other ____ Consult communication disorders
CONTROL OF PAIN: ____ Acute ____ Chronic RELATED TO:	Relief of pain: Self-regulate control measures	___ Report pain ___ Report responses to treatments	Observe/record effects ____ Teach: ____ Consult clinical nurse specialist re:

(continued)

NURSING ACTION PLAN: IMMEDIATE *(continued)*

# AND DATE PLUS SELF-CARE DEFICIT ACTUAL/ POTENTIAL (PROBLEM)	GOAL/TIME TO BE COMPLETED	PATIENT/ CAREGIVER ACTIONS	NURSING ACTIONS
CONTROL OF ELIMINATION ____ Bladder program RELATED TO:	Self-managed continence	Report: ____ Need to void ____ Need to be catheterized ____ Accidents	____ Initiate bladder program: ____ Begin teaching:
CONTROL OF ELIMINATION Bowel program RELATED TO:	Self-managed continence	Report: ____ Need to defecate ____ Effect of program ____ Accident	____ Initiate bowel program: ____ Begin teaching:
MANAGING DIET/INTAKE RE: ____ Eating ____ Self-feeding ____ Tube feeding ____ Swallowing fluids: ____ Oral ____ Intravenous RELATED TO:	Follow prescribed diet, manage self-feeding	Select/eat appropriate food, drink adequate fluids	Observe intake: Provide: ____ Set-up ____ Feed ____ Floor tray ____ Cafeteria ____ Refer for feeding program ____ Initiate swallowing program

(continued)

NURSING ACTION PLAN: IMMEDIATE *(continued)*

# AND DATE PLUS SELF-CARE DEFICIT ACTUAL/ POTENTIAL (PROBLEM)	GOAL/TIME TO BE COMPLETED	PATIENT/ CAREGIVER ACTIONS	NURSING ACTIONS
SAFETY PRECAUTIONS OR RISK RE: ____ Allergic reactions ____ Breathing control ____ Ventilator ____ Choking/aspiration ____ Falls ____ Wandering ____ Performance of skin care ____ Prevention ____ Management ____ Smoking in bed RELATED TO:	No reaction No falls or injuries No skin breakdown Maintains Manages protective measures Refrain from or safe control of smoking	Report risk factors, symptoms Observe safety precautions re mobility Observe risk sites, report symptoms/signs ____ Not smoke in bed ____ Use robot smoker ____ Take precautions	____ Document: ____ Notify physician ____ Monitor activities until safe conduct is evident ____ Restraint, posey vest ____ Lap board (circle) ____ Red flag ____ Check pressure sites at least weekly ____ Begin program ____ Instruct about fire ____ Observe smoking behavior ____ Restrict: ____ Matches ____ Cigarettes ____ Provide robot smoker
GENERAL: Control over self-care system: ____ None ____ Inadequate ____ Incomplete Related to ____ Hospitalization ____ Condition (specify) ____ Treatment (specify)	Restoration of control over self-care by self/dependent caregiver by discharge	Listen, learn, ask questions, ask for help as needed, cooperate	Teach, explain procedures, activity schedule, guide, support as needed, do for, assist as appropriate Document actions/responses

NURSE'S SIGNATURE   DATE

NURSING DIAGNOSIS:
ADMISSION/DISCHARGE (circle appropriate one)

SELF-CARE REQUISITES	MET	NOT MET	SELF-CARE LIMITATIONS	ABILITIES

Met: Y: Yes
      N/A: Not applicable
 	
Not Met: P: Partial
         C: Complete
         U: Unidentified
			Knowledge, Judgment, Physical Abilities and Willingness
			
			REASONS WHY NOT TO DO
			Include conditioning factors
			Describe disability effects only once unless specific aspect
				Assets Operative and Helpful in Meeting Demands

UNIVERSALS
Number:
 	
  Maintain sufficient
  intake of air				

____ Breathe ____ Cough Balance rest and activity				
____ Mobility ____ Control energy/fatigue ____ Pace self ____ Care re elimination				
____ Bladder program ____ Bowel program Intake				
____ Food/diet ____ Fluids ____ Eat ____ Swallow				

NURSING DIAGNOSIS:ADMISSION/DISCHARGE (continued)

SELF-CARE REQUISITES	MET	NOT MET	SELF-CARE LIMITATIONS	ABILITIES
Prevent Hazards ____ Allergy ____ Call for help/nurse ____ Control behavior ____ Electrical equipment ____ Falls ____ Infection ____ Seizures ____ Skin breakdown ____ Smoking **Balance Solitude and Social Interaction**			Secondary to: ____ Age 70+ ____ Poor judgment ____ Impulsive	
Normalcy ____ Communication ____ Self-image ____ Sexuality ____ Usual self-care hygiene ____ Bathe ____ Groom ____ Monitor self (body functions)				
DEVELOPMENTAL Maturational:				
Situational:				
____ Adjustment to disability ____ Family adjustment				

(continued)

NURSING DIAGNOSIS: ADMISSION/DISCHARGE *(continued)*

SELF-CARE REQUISITES	MET	NOT MET	SELF-CARE LIMITATIONS	ABILITIES
HEALTH DEVIATION				
Knowledge				
____ Condition				
____ Diagnostic procedure				
____ Treatment				
____ Hospital				
____ Rehab in general				
Performance				
____ Monitor condition/treatment				
____ Carry out treatment				
____ Self-medication				
____ Use appliance/equip.				

Summary: Mark Below as Applicable
NUMBER OF SELF-CARE REQUISITES: SELF-CARE CAPABILITIES

___ Met: ____ Future Potential Deficit   ____ Developed
____ Unmet: ____ Not Operable   ____ Operable
____ New   ____ Old   ____ Not Adequate   ____ Adequate
____ Temporary   ____ Permanent   ____ No Potential for Development/
____ Complete   ____ Partial   Redevelopment
                          ____ Extensive   ____ Limited Potential for Development/
                          ____ Moderate   Redevelopment
                          ____ Minimal (1 or 2)

FAMILY/CAREGIVER COMMENTS re: above problem number

NURSING ACTION PLAN: CONTINUING
(MUST BE COMPLETED WITHIN FIRST WEEK OF ADMISSION)

NUMBER & DATE: SELF-CARE DEFICIT ACTUAL/ POTENTIAL PROBLEM	GOAL/TIME TO BE COMPLETED	PATIENT/ CAREGIVER ACTIONS	NURSING ACTIONS
USE OF KNOWLEDGE ____ Rehabilitation ____ Health condition management ____ arthritis ____ drug control ____ head injury ____ pain ____ spinal injury ____ stroke ____ surgery: ____ neurology ____ *other:* RELATED TO:	Verbalizes/ demonstrates basic knowledge, performs essential care measures	Attend classes	____ Explain basic rehabilitation ____ Begin disability education program ____ Consult clinical nurse specialist for: ____ Consult rehab nurse for:
CONTROL BEHAVIOR RELATED TO:	Adequate control of:		Initiate the following
COPE WITH DISABILITY: ____ self ____ family RELATED TO:	Use appropriate method as prescribed		Consult
CONTROL/ MANAGE MOBILITY: RELATED TO:	Use appropriate method as prescribed		Assist to:
SLEEP/REST RELATED TO:			

(continued)

NURSING ACTION PLAN: CONTINUING *(continued)*

NUMBER & DATE: SELF-CARE DEFICIT ACTUAL/ POTENTIAL PROBLEM	GOAL/TIME TO BE COMPLETED	PATIENT/ CAREGIVER ACTIONS	NURSING ACTIONS
TO PERFORM MEASURES: ____ Bathing: ____ bed ____ shower ____ other: ____ Dressing: ____ upper extremity ____ lower extremity ____ hose ____ shoes ____Use appliances ____ razor ____ dryer ____ braces/ splints ____ other			
TO MANAGE TREATMENT ____ Self-medication ____ Wound care ____ Other RELATED TO:			
TO PREVENT POTENTIAL: ____ Infection ____ Urinary ____ Other ____ Seizures RELATED TO:	No infection, follows safe procedures Minimal to no seizures, take appropriate precautions	Take precautions, report signs and symptoms; follow proper care procedures Report prodromal symptoms, if any; take medication as prescribed	____Observe for signs ____ Maintain universal precautions ____ Consult infection control nurse ____ Monitor ____ Maintain medication schedule ____ Take protective measures

NURSING ACTION PLAN: CONTINUING *(continued)*

DEPENDENT CARE DEFICIT

_____
TO MANAGE

RELATED TO:

PLANS/GOALS DISCUSSED WITH PATIENT/FAMILY ____ Y   ____ N

_____   _____
PATIENT / FAMILY SIGNATURE   DATE

_____   _____
NURSE SIGNATURE   DATE

SELF-CARE ACTIVITIES FLOWSHEET

Code Each Activity:

NA: NOT APPLICABLE	A: ASSISTED (partially)	CODE FOR	Code for each week
I: INDEPENDENT	D: DEPENDENT	"KNOWS"	(place an asterisk by
E: INDEPENDENT/	U: UNIDENTIFIED	C: COMPLETE	activity if progress
EQUIPMENT		P: PARTIAL	note written). If no
S: SUPERVISION			changes, write "no change" vertically.

Date   1st wk of Admission   Discharge

ACTIVITY	ASSISTANCE/ EQUIPMENT NEEDED	KNOWS		DOES							KNOWS		DOES	
		Y	N	Y	N	1	2	3	4	5	Y	N	Y	N
APPLIANCES														
1. Communication														
2. Dentures														
3. Glasses (eye)														
4. Hearing aid														
5. Splint/brace														
6. Prosthesis														
ELIMINATION														
7. Bladder program														
8. Bowel program														
GROOMING														
8. Dressing—upper														
9. Dressing—lower														
10. Hair—comb/wash														
HYGIENE														
11. Bath-shower-tub														
12. Teeth														
13. Shave/feet/nails														
14. Perineal														
INTAKE														
15. Eat/feed self														
16. Fluids/food/drink														
17. Swallowing prog.														
MOBILITY														
18. Ambulate														
19. WC/gurney														
20. Transfer to/from chair														
21. Positioning														

SELF-CARE ACTIVITIES FLOWSHEET *(continued)*

ACTIVITY	ASSISTANCE/ EQUIPMENT NEEDED	KNOWS		DOES		1	2	3	4	5	KNOWS		DOES	
		Y	N	Y	N	1	2	3	4	5	Y	N	Y	N
MOBILITY *(continued)* 22. Raises														
23. Turning														
SAFETY-MGT. 24. Call nurse														
25. Control behavior														
26. Electrical equipment														
27. Fall prevention														
28. Smoking														
29. Skin protection														
TREATMENTS 30. Heat/cold														
31. Self-medicate														
32. Wound care														
33. Other														
TOTAL: Applicable activities														

SUMMARY:
ADMISSION TOTAL BY CATEGORY: I:____ E:____ S____ A:____ D:____ NA/U:____
DISCHARGE TOTAL BY CATEGORY: I:____ E:____ S____ A:____ D:____ NA/U:____

WK/ADM \ 1 \ 2 \ 3 \ 4 \ 5 \ 6 \ DISCHARGE
PATIENT CLASSIFICATION:
MANAGEMENT OF HEALTH DEVIATION PROGRAM:

	KNOWS		DOES			KNOWS		DOES	
	Y	N	Y	N		Y	N	Y	N
34. Arthritis									
35. Pain management									
36. Spinal injury									
37. Stroke/brain injury									
38. Other									

FAMILY/CAREGIVER'S ABILITIES/ LIMITATIONS ABOVE: (Give number of activity, date, note)

_____   _____
Nurse's signature: Date

Philosophical Statements, Standards, and Forms From a Community Health Setting

T his appendix contains philosophical statements, a nursing practice standard, assessment standards, and documentation forms originally developed by a community health nursing service (the Vancouver Health Department in Vancouver, Canada) that were used by nurses in the home care nursing program and the prevention program. Note the theoretical consistency between the standards, the statements, and the forms.

The appendix first presents extracts from the nursing practice standards and the philosophical statement. The standard states that the major focus of nursing is the promotion of health-related self-care. Self-care is further elaborated on in the philosophy, which states that self-care is a requirement common to all human beings and that self-care actions are deliberate and are linked to ethnic and cultural customs.

The assessment standards illustrate operationalization of this philosophical statement and standard. Extracts from the assessment standards pertaining to mothers in the 0- to 28-day postpartum period for the general population and as specified for the Vietnamese population are

AUTHORS' NOTE: The forms and extracts in the appendix come from unpublished documents of the Vancouver Health Department, Vancouver, Canada. Materials reprinted courtesy of the Vancouver/ Richmond Health Board.

provided. Note that nurses are directed to explore actions to be taken to meet self-care requisites and capability to meet those requisites within the context of the current conditioning factors. One conditioning factor is related to health state (being in the 0- to 28-day postpartum period); the other is related to sociocultural beliefs.

The first extract from the documentation system is a form that provides a means for documenting information about the capability of the mother to meet her self-care requisites. A second form provides a means for documenting information about self-care capabilities (agency).

Philosophical Statements and Nursing Practice Standard

The following are excerpts from "Philosophy of Community Health Nursing":

Nursing provides services within a multicultural community to people at all stages of development and in all health states. The particular service that nursing provides is an assisting one. That assistance can be offered through episodic or continual contact. What is accomplished directly or indirectly through nursing is an enhanced capacity for self-care by individuals, families and communities of persons so that they can achieve and maintain optimal health.

Assistance offered by community health nurses is based on the belief that:

1. Requirements for self-care are common to all human beings and are learned within the context of social groups by communication and human interaction.
2. Some requirements for self-care result from illness related limitations which make self-care difficult or impossible.
3. Self-care actions are deliberate actions learned and performed to meet and know needs for care.
4. People's beliefs and values about health and self-care actions are inseparably linked to ethnic and cultural customs.

The following is an excerpt from "Standards for Nursing Practice":

The major focus of nursing is the promotion of health related self-care. This is accomplished by working with individuals, families, and community groups.

Excerpt From "Assessment Standards"

Actions to Be Taken by Client (Self-Care Demand)	Knowledge, Skill, Ability to Take Action (Self-Care Agency)	Sociocultural Factors	Nursing Actions
Maintains a balance between solitude and social interaction Incorporates time for self into daily routine Incorporates time for significant others into daily routine Balances need for social contact with need for quiet times Takes action to reestablish relationship as a couple Obtains adequate support from significant others Other	Organizational skill Knowledge, mobility, energy, and motivation to take action Ability to perform in more than one role.	Traditionally, the Vietnamese family would have at least one other woman in the home, the mother-in-law. She would do all the cooking and housework, and much of the infant care in the first 30 days. She is also the one to ensure that the woman is complying with the dietary restriction and mobility restrictions. In Canada, if this is not possible, the husband will usually help out, but the postpartum mother often has to be more active than she thinks she should be. It is very lonely for her if she does not have a woman's company. When there isn't a supportive female in the house, her husband fulfills this role	Be aware of the cultural need of a supportive female in the home and recognize the impact of no other woman in the home Recognize potential for loneliness and isolation

Documentation Forms

Assessment of Self-Care Requisites

NAME_____CONTINUING CARE #_____

CODE:

✔ = No Nursing Invervention   D = Deficit   P = Potential Deficit   NA = Not Assessed

A. UNIVERSAL SELF-CARE REQUISITES	DATE/CODE/ INITIAL	B. DEVELOPMENTAL SELF-CARE REQUISITES	DATE/CODE/ INITIAL
1. Maintenance of sufficient intake of air		1. Provides conditions that promote/support development	
2. Maintenance of sufficient intake of fluid		2. Prevents/overcomes conditions that affect development	
3. Maintenance of sufficient intake of food		C. HEALTH DEVIATION SELF-CARE REQUISITES	
4. Provision of care associated with elimination		1. Seeks and secures assistance (medical/ community resources)	
5. Maintenance of sleep/ activity balance		2. Attends to effects of pathological state	
6. Maintenance of social/ solitude balance		3. Carries out prescribed measures	
7. Prevention of hazards		4. Regulates deleterious effects of prescribed measures	
8. Promotion of normalcy			

(continued)

Overview Assessment of Self-Care Agency

CODE: ✔ = Adequate   N = Not Adequate   D = Declining   NA = Not Assessed

SELF-CARE AGENCY (Self-Care Capabilities/ Limitations)	DATE/CODE/INITIAL	DEPENDENT CARE AGENCY DATE/CODE/INITIAL
Capabilities of knowing		
Capabilities of decision making		
Capabilities of acting		

Materials From
Acute Care Settings

This appendix contains sample materials extracted from the clinical information systems of an acute care setting. In acute care, identifying the specific information at a particular point in time is important. Staff in these settings cannot deal with the whole scope of variables that have been identified as of interest to nursing but must decide which self-care requisites, conditioning factors, or particular features of self-care agency are the most significant features in a situation at the time.

Excerpt From the Data Collection System
in an Acute Care Setting

The following items have been excerpted from the data collection system in an acute care setting. Note that along with identifying data items, the purpose for collecting the item has also been identified.

Items included in neonatal intensive care unit data collection tool:

Maintaining a balance between rest and activity

Activity: ____ Normal

                                 ____ Active

                                 ____ Minimal

                                 ____ Hyperactive

                                 ____ Irritable

Cry: ____ Normal

                                 ____ High pitched

                                 ____ Other (describe)

Following individual patient developmental regime ____ Yes____ No

Meeting self-care requisite requires the assistance of:

____ Caregiver

____ Nurse

____ Both

Maintaining a balance between solitude and social interaction

Support system available ____ Mother

                                 ____ Father

                                 ____ Significant other

                                 ____ None

Following individual patient developmental regime ____ Yes____ No

Observed parent/child bonding: (Describe)

Extract From Plan of Care for Patients Undergoing
a Cardiovascular Surgical Procedure, Demonstrating
Direction From Self-Care Deficit Nursing Theory

Focus of Concern/ Nursing Diagnosis	Goals	Patient/Family Actions	Nursing Actions	Comments
Limited exercise of self-care agency because of present health state post "surgical procedure" Particular concerns: Possible bleeding Possible infection Vascular injury	Meet components of therapeutic self-care demand re: Prevention of hazards Maintenance of sufficient intake of air Maintenance of balance between rest and activity Promotion of normalcy	Not flex R/L leg/arm while arterial/venous catheters are in place and for 6 hours after removal Read and verbalize understanding of post sheath removal written instructions Report wet/warm sensation around R/L groin/arm Report numbness or tingling in R/L foot/arm	Continuously monitor leads Obtain initial 12-lead ECG and PRN Monitor ST segment for depression or T-wave inversion and document Monitor BP, P, R every 15 minutes × 4 hours, then every 30 minutes × 2 hours, and then every 1 hour and prn.	

Extract From Standards of Care
Demonstrating Use of Self-Care Deficit
Nursing Theory in an Acute Care Setting

GENERIC ISOLATION STANDARD OF CARE

Purpose: Protection from hazards.

Focus of Concern: To protect patients, health care workers, and visitors from communicable disease.

Nursing Actions:

1. Identify the specific type of isolation required based on suspected organisms and mode of transmission.
2. Transfer patient to appropriate room if required.
3. Instruct patient on nature of isolation and patient/family role.
4. Complete appropriate documentation: patient record, infection control department
5. Redesign patient care plan:

   a. Identify impact of isolation technique on actions required to meet patient's therapeutic self-care demand.

   b. Assess the patient's capabilities to meet therapeutic self-care demand.

   c. Develop appropriate care plan.

Note: Particular self-care requisites of concern include:

1. Provision of care related to processes of elimination
2. Maintenance of a balance between rest and activity and between solitude and social interaction
3. Promotion of normalcy
4. Overcoming of factors that interfere with development

Quality Control

Patient Outcomes

Q uality control is concerned with standards of care and practice: the structures, the processes, and the outcomes of nursing. This chapter focuses on outcomes, the difficulties in defining nursing outcomes, and how self-care deficit nursing theory (Orem, 1995) provides a basis for identifying nursing outcomes. A framework for categorizing nursing outcomes based on the theory is proposed. Examples using the theory for determining nursing outcomes in rehabilitation and acute care nursing including use of a patient classification system are given. In addition, a framework for examining nursing outcomes in terms of individuals, populations, and nursing administration is presented.

A Perspective on Quality

Definition

Quality can be defined as an attribute, an acquired trait, or an accomplishment or as excellence of a characteristic (*Webster's New Collegiate Dictionary*, 1953, p. 691). Quality, as generally understood, refers to excellence in one or more attributes or characteristics. Control of quality in a health care organization seeks to meet established goals and obtain outcomes of concern to the organization as a whole and to its processes. Today, many factors relating to patients, the services provided, and operations supportive to them within organizations are being examined. Evaluation of quality necessitates assurance of available data about all aspects of the organization.

Issues in Measuring Quality

Much has been written about ways to measure quality and to improve on the quality of care for different types of patients and health care organizations. Donabedian (1968) established a commonly accepted framework for measuring quality: structure, process, and outcomes. *Structure* is concerned with the type of organizational framework established, governance, medical staff, policies and procedures, types and mix of personnel, staffing methods, standards of various types, and so forth. *Process* refers to the numbers and types of actions taken in encounters between patients and providers of care, the rules and practices. *Outcomes* are the end results of the actions taken in terms of patients, personnel performance, and organizational performance in light of established goals and standards.

Donabedian's three factors have been addressed in a variety of studies. Pierce (1997) considered all three factors and focused on outcome indicators. She also suggested that nursing care delivery systems be examined in relation to clinical nursing studies. An American Nurses Association publication (*An Emerging Framework*, 1995) presented a variety of nursing classification databases that are being developed and tested: diagnoses, interventions, outcomes, and other factors. The need for a common language to describe nursing was recognized. Meisenheimer (1997) presented what it takes to develop and conduct quality improvement programs and described processes toward that end.

Structure, as discussed by Alexander, Bourgeois, and Goodman (1994), focused on shared governance and total quality improvement. Deming's principles for empowering employees in decision making were seen as process variables. Professional provider-client elements identified included (a) utilization of health care services, (b) clinical status indicators, (c) severity of health problem, (d) adherence to recommended care regimen, and (e) satisfaction with care (Carter & Kulbok, 1995). Blegen, Goode, and Reed (1998) studied the effect of registered nurse (RN) skill mix and hours of care (structural variables) on patient outcomes. They found that the more hours of RN care given, the fewer the adverse outcomes—medication errors (process variable), falls, decubiti, and complaints from patients and families. Doswell (1989) cited outcomes in terms of the behavioral, physiological, perceptual, and attitudinal dimensions and suggested that selection of criteria to measure outcomes "requires a clear set of standards of practice" (p. 21). (Standards are discussed in the next chapter.)

Patient-Related Outcomes

Commonly accepted outcomes for health care systems are mortality; discharge disposition—death, return home, or nursing home placement; length of stay; readmission; total number of infections; total number of respiratory complications; and life-threatening complications. Some, such as Daubert (1979), identify outcomes by level of care—from acute nonchronic to end-stage illness. Edwardson (1988) listed types of outcomes in terms of patient response. These include mortality, ability to work or perform daily activities, fulfillment of other regular social roles, sexual functioning, and avoidance of readmission to the hospital. Edwardson also noted difficulty in sorting out medical outcomes from outcomes of other health services or organizational factors such as personnel policies, management practices, and stability of nursing staff.

General patient outcomes as defined by Brett (1989) include measured changes in behavior; any alteration in clinical health status; patient knowledge and understanding of disease or treatment; functional health status; patient satisfaction; psychoemotional health status; perceptions of patient, family, nurses, and physicians; disposition of patients on discharge; negative results such as complications; discharge readiness of the patient; compliance with the health care regimen; and appearance of the patient. Other outcomes Brett listed include days at home versus days in hospital, readmissions to hospital, length of stay, mortality rates, and costs of care.

Patient satisfaction as an outcome variable in any form of health care delivery is frequently cited in outcome studies. Avis (1994) noted that there is no established theoretical framework for understanding the determinant of patient satisfaction in relation to treatment effectiveness. The use of patient satisfaction as a variable is fraught with problems, even though every effort is made to control them. Reasons might be hesitation to be critical because of fear that the service might be needed again or because options to go elsewhere may be limited. The response may reflect the mood or condition the person is in at the time of response or the distortion of a whole episode of care by one unpleasant incident. Satisfaction with services may come from the knowledge that a variety of care is readily available, accessible, attentive, and affordable. Some may not be so concerned about who provides the care so long as they personally feel that the care provided is adequate to meet their needs and is there when needed. The patient may equate comfort with quality, not knowing the nature of the service required in the situation. A popular assumption is that health care will be provided one way or another and should be the best possible.

Brook, McGlynn, and Cleary (1996) suggested that process outcomes may be more sensitive measures of quality than outcome data because poor outcomes do not occur every time there is an error in provision of care. Outcomes may be strongly influenced by differences in patient characteristics. In view of this, both process and outcomes need to be addressed to prevent deterioration in quality over the long run.

Issues Related to Indicators of Quality of Nursing

The particular problem in nursing is to identify indicators of quality of nursing as distinguished from those of other health care disciplines and the field in general. In reports on patient outcomes, Marek (1989a) noted that no current database clearly reflects the status of clients as a result of receiving nursing. This concern is reiterated in the 1996 Institute of Medicine study on nurse staffing (Wunderlich, Sloan, & Davis, 1996). In the following studies, no consistent commonly accepted model or framework is evident as a basis for identifying outcomes specific to nursing.

Marek (1989b) reiterated many of the general outcomes previously cited and added broad general indicators such as physiological, psychological, functional, and behavioral factors, knowledge, patient satisfaction, safety, and resolution of nursing diagnoses. Gillis (1995) stated that nursing outcomes include but are not limited to lifestyle behaviors, knowledge, well-being, quality of life, coping behavior, attitudes, and values. The nursing role is to focus on positive lifestyle changes rather than specific behavioral changes because the global outcome is health promotion: that is, self-responsibility for health—making choices consistent with a healthy lifestyle. Zander (1995) cited four clinical outcomes: health outcomes, knowledge outcomes, activity (physical/role function), and absence of complications. She noted these might be called "products" in industrial engineering terms and can be achieved through collaborative care by using process protocols—critical paths or care maps. The foregoing outcomes relate to the standards for patient education developed by the Joint Commission on Accreditation of Health Care Organizations. Process standards are included. The Joint Commission standards are based on the 1975 Patients' Bill of Rights, which emphasizes the patient's right to information about his or her diagnosis, treat-

TABLE 8.1 Outcome Variables Identified in Literature Review

Marek (1989b)	Gillis (1995)	Zander (1995)	ANA (1995)
Physiological	Lifestyle behavior	Health	Nosocomial infection
Psychological	Knowledge	Knowledge	Patient injury rate
Functional	Well-being	Activity	Patient satisfaction
Behavioral	Quality of life	Absence of	Maintenance of skin
Knowledge	Coping behavior	complications	integrity
Patient satisfaction	Attitudes		Nursing satisfaction
Safety	Steady status		Mix of RN, LPN,
Resolution of			assistants
nursing diagnosis			Total hours of
			nursing care

ment, and prognosis needed to make informed decisions (Association of Operating Nurses, 1996).

Process variables are nursing actions relating outcomes to predetermined factors such as client behavioral change or acquisition of knowledge or skills (Gillis, 1995). Though many outcomes may be predetermined, others may be unintended or unexpected. Moreover, a steady, constant status may be as desirable an outcome as a change in status (Gillis, 1995). Recent efforts to classify nursing-sensitive outcomes have attempted to standardize the language and articulate nursing diagnoses and nursing interventions. A nursing-sensitive outcome is defined as "a variable patient or family caregiver state, behavior, or perception that is responsive to nursing intervention and conceptualized at middle levels of abstraction (e.g., mobility level, nutritional status, health attitudes" (Maas, Johnson, & Morehead, 1996, p. 296). Indicators may be identified for lower level (more specific) states.

The American Nurses Association recognizes seven quality indicators: (a) nosocomial infections, (b) patient injury rate, (c) patient satisfaction, (d) maintenance of skin integrity, (e) nursing staff satisfaction, (f) mix of RNs, licensed practical nurses (LPNs), and unlicensed nursing personnel, and (g) total nursing care hours per day (Canavan, 1996). When looking at the variables to predict nursing costs per diagnosis-related group (DRG), Grohn, Myers, and McSweeney (1996) found that the determinant for nursing must rely on the functional needs of the patient.

From all of this, it is apparent that *nursing has no consistent identifiable mental model or framework* by which to determine and evaluate the quality of nursing care. The variables identified in the foregoing studies are summarized in Table 8.1.

Self-Care Deficit Nursing Theory:
A Framework for Specifying Outcomes

A definitive mental model or framework for nursing helps to establish and clarify the structure, processes, and outcomes to be achieved through nursing. According to Orem's (1995) general theory of nursing, the object of nurses who engage in the practice of nursing is persons who seek and can benefit from nursing because of existent or predicted health-derived or health-related self-care or dependent care deficits. Furthermore, the object of nursing administration is "the definable but changing population of persons for whom a legally constituted enterprise ensures the continuing availability and actual provision of nursing" (Orem, 1989, pp. 55-56). Two types of nursing administrative actions are concerned with the populations served: (a) the continuous description of the population from a nursing perspective and (b) the continuous calculation of what is required to provide nursing to populations now and at a future time (Orem, 1989). These entail establishing, providing, and evaluating the processes and outcomes of nursing.

Quality care requires nursing to attain particular goals by (a) establishing ways to ensure that nursing is available and provided to meet existent or predicted health-derived or health-related self-care or dependent care deficits of a definitive but changing population of persons served or to be served; and (b) establishing means to evaluate whether self/dependent care deficits are overcome, self/dependent care capabilities are maintained and/or increased, and factors affecting both are controlled as much as possible.

Nursing outcomes or results of nursing systems can be defined in both general and specific terms. They must concern therapeutic self-care demands being known and met: that therapeutic self/dependent care is produced at definitive periods or sequences in time and that self/dependent care agency is regulated—protected, increased, and exercised. Self-management is considered in terms of establishing and maintaining a self-care system and the adequacy of that system in relation to the system of daily living. With dependent care, the system of care should be adequately managed and incorporated into daily family life. In the production design model in Chapter 6, broad general health goals of life, health, well-being, and effective living are listed. Nursing and self/dependent care are essential to these goals. More specifically, these goals relate to the health focus of the following health situations: (a) life cycle adjustments in promotion and maintenance of health and well-being, prevention of illness, and effective living; (b) recovery from illness or injury; (c) regulation or cure of the condition (including prevention of complications); (d) rehabilitation/restoration; (e) stabilization of the condition; and (f) comfort as much as possible in all situations, including dying (Orem, 1995).

Not listed as solely nursing goals are reducing costs, a concern of health care system payers, including patients. Meeting this goal would entail, for example, controlling the length of stay in the hospital and preventing readmissions and emergency room visits. All add to the expense. Costs are relevant to all health care disciplines, not just nursing. Reduction of expenses is an administrative concern, not primarily a clinical one.

Orem (1990) more precisely identified the results of nursing with respect to patients. These are

1. Knowledge of therapeutic self-care demands and regulation of the values of each component in relation to human functioning and development
2. Effective meeting of components of therapeutic self-care demands in time-specific sequence
3. Regulation of the exercise of self-care or dependent care agency

For the nurse, results relate to the nurse's knowledge and judgment about the need to alter the form of the nursing system—whether to continue or to move to a dependent care or self-care system (Orem, 1990). The desired end product is an adequate functional self-care system or a dependent care system so that a nursing system is no longer needed.

The practical results to be achieved through self/dependent care and/or nursing are to

1. Increase, maintain, and protect self-care agency
2. Overcome self-care deficits by
   a. Meeting self-care requisites both quantitatively and qualitatively
   b. Ascertaining whether self/dependent care is adequate to continuously meet therapeutic self-care demand in that the required health care prescribed and needed is provided
3. Coordinate self/dependent care and nursing with other health services; this includes those aspects of health state under nursing jurisdiction to be monitored and regulated at an optimum level given the particular situation

The study best known for its reliability and validity of criterion measures for nursing-sensitive patient outcomes based on Orem's theory is the work of Horn and Swain (1977), carried out in the 1970s. Current writings by Brett (1989) and Marek (1989a) continue to recognize the contribution of this work on nursing outcomes. Another early study based on Orem's theory cited several specific self-care criteria as valid (Gallant & McLane, 1979). More recent work by Lee and Dean (1995) used Holzemer's (1992) model of patient outcomes research. This model addresses the patient/client, the provider, and the setting in terms of the inputs (structural elements), processes, and patient/client outcomes in relation to health and well-being and self-care skills. Kitson (1986) used Orem's types of nursing systems to define levels of dependency—wholly compensatory, partly compensatory, and educative-supportive—and related them to two types of nursing measures. These were tested on a geriatric patient population. In a more recent study of patient outcomes, self-care deficit nursing theory was used as an organizer in relation to nursing diagnosis and the Nursing Intervention Classification (NIC) categories. These outcomes are profiled under six domains: basic physiologic, complex physiologic, behavioral, family, health system, and safety. The particular variables under each domain are not clearly identified in the self-care deficit nursing theory context. The majority appear to relate to the self-care requisites and basic conditioning factors (Micek et al., 1996). Three major levels of care identified are (a) "restoring the patient to an improved condition," (b) "maintaining the patient's current condition," and (c) "increasing self care agency" (Micek et al., 1996, p. 32).

An Example From Rehabilitation

A group of nurse managers and nurse case managers in a rehabilitation hospital were interviewed to determine what they would look for in terms of outcomes of care, particularly nursing, as a legitimate reason for making a home visit on every patient discharged from the hospital. The responses given were analyzed and organized from the self-care deficit nursing theory perspective. These rehabilitation nurses, many of whom had previously been exposed to the theory, were well aware of the adjustments necessary in self-care as a consequence of a disability. See Appendix 8A for a summary of the nurses' responses. Their replies were primarily concerned with self/dependent care agency: self-care operations and power components, what persons were now able to do or not do in the home environment, and some basic conditioning factors (BCFs). The information given does not cover the potential range of outcomes from the self-care deficit nursing theory perspective.

Rehabilitation is a long-term process. Rehabilitation nursing is concerned with assisting persons with physical disabilities to develop an adequate self-care system to meet universal, developmental, and health deviation self-care requisites as changes occur over time to promote and maintain health and to incorporate the self-care system into a system of daily living. Numerous complex adjustments may be necessary that place demands on the physically challenged individual and family or caregiver, if needed. Developing an adequate self-care system includes incorporating prescriptions of physicians and therapists, making adjustments in the social and physical environment, incorporating self/dependent care systems into the system of daily living, and appropriately utilizing and accommodating to the health care system.

The rehabilitation nurses' responses tended to reflect concerns about problems and outcomes that might occur both on immediate hospital discharge and over the long term (see Appendix 8A). Concerns of insurance companies also mentioned consisted of potential early problems relating to self/dependent care agency such as inadequacy in self-care operations: noncompliance, alcohol or drug abuse, poor care, and lack of or poor family support and care. From the technical knowledge perspective, the types of problems mentioned were lack of knowledge about home care needs, such as lack of understanding about the need to catheterize regularly, to turn, and to do "raises" to prevent pressure sores. From the basic conditioning factors aspect, potential complications cited may result from inadequacy in self-care, such as resistant urinary tract infections, skin breakdown, bowel impaction, injury related to falls, and dislocation of a new joint. Other concerns were a possible recurrent stroke or seizure and dysfunctional families. Health care system factors included inadequate follow-up and a length of stay too short for patients and families to absorb the important aspects of the care required, so that some parts were overlooked or forgotten.

Predominant nursing concerns are about what patients and caregivers are doing to regulate and protect altered body functions and structures associated with the type of disability and certain basic conditioning factors. Basic questions nurses must answer are:

1. What required care in whole or part must be managed on a continuing daily basis and/or periodically?
2. Is it being provided, and if so, how well?
3. By whom—patient, dependent care agent, nurse, or some combination?
4. If not provided and/or not adequate, why not? How best can the required care be provided and ensured?

A clinical management problem is to prioritize the types of actions essential to ensure performance of at least a minimal safe level in exercise of self-care by the patient and/or caregiver in the least time. Hopefully, some assurance of consistency in performance of patients/caregivers and continuance after hospital discharge, either on their own or with nursing supervision through home health care, needs to be considered. Another objective is to prevent readmissions for complications arising from failure in self-care. In other words, considerable attention and effort on the part of nursing and other health care services, such as physical, occupational, and respiratory therapies and social work, must be made to ensure that the schedule of patient activities fits in with the patient's goals, wishes, pattern of daily living, resources, and environment if a therapeutic regimen is to be maintained. Interdisciplinary collaboration is needed with the patient and/or caregiver to ensure that a workable acceptable system of daily care is worked out and followed.

Self-Care Deficit Nursing Theory Outcome Categories

A theoretical framework incorporating the variables and their subsets is proposed as a practical means for answering the foregoing questions and making judgments about nursing processes and outcomes. An outline for identifying categories for nursing outcomes based on the self-care deficit theory of nursing can be seen in Table 8.2.

From analysis of the nurses' statements about outcomes looked for in rehabilitation (Appendix 8A) and from general experience in nursing, outcome categories based on the self-care deficit nursing theory could easily be developed and organized. Note that Categories 1 through 4—self/dependent care systems, therapeutic self-care demand, self-care agency, and dependent care—focus on patients/clients and/or caregivers—their status, capabilities, and actions performed. The fifth category, the basic conditioning factors that affect self-care, comprises the factors most frequently cited in outcomes studies. Nursing is involved only when self-dependent care is affected or needed to regulate them. This often is done in conjunction with other health care disciplines. The last two categories focus on nursing. These concern what is directly regulated through nursing in relation to patient/client actions to control basic conditioning factors affecting the self/dependent care system. These categories have not been tested and validated through research. It is work that needs to be done. Nurses familiar with the theory and aided by appropriate documentation tools can gather this type of information. See Chapter 7, Appendix 7A, for examples of means of gathering some of this information in a rehabilitation situation.

■ *Sample Forms for Evaluating Nursing Outcomes*

The rehabilitation forms in Appendix 7A address many nursing outcomes categories outlined in Table 8.2. They focus in on the nursing component of an interdisciplinary health service. Nursing follows through by assisting patients with many adjustments in self-care activities prescribed by various therapies— occupational, physical, speech, respiratory, and so forth. Two forms, "Nursing Diagnosis" and the "Nursing/Self-Care Activities Flowsheet," are designed to show change or maintenance of status in terms of managing various aspects of self-care. The nursing diagnosis form lists self-care requisites of most frequent concern and whether they are met at time of admission and again at time of discharge. It includes the reasons why in terms of self-care limitations and capabilities for meeting therapeutic self-care demand. The number of requisites met and unmet can be quantitatively summarized. How well, qualitatively, also can be identified in terms of not meeting them, partly meeting them, or com- pletely meeting them. The form includes some characteristics of self-care requisites, such as whether they are new or old and whether they are temporary and may or may not require attention. It provides an opportunity to list potential future deficits and to describe the status of (changes in) self-care agency in terms of the power components and self-care operations—their development, oper- ability, and adequacy. Brief space also is provided on the forms to indicate the status of the dependent care agent with regard to managing or co-managing specific requisites. These are identified by problem number.

The Nursing Self-Care Activities Flowsheet gets down to specific action demands with regard to level of dependency in the activity. The levels are "independent," "independent with equipment," "supervision only," "assisted (partly)," and "dependent." In addition, for each activity, whether the individual knows what to do and how, in whole or in part, should be identified. This is foundational to taking an action. Many rehabilitation patients physically may not be able to perform an action but can make decisions and direct another in the process. On this form a person's status each week in the course of hospitali- zation can be noted. If data from groups of patients with a similar type of disability are analyzed, certain features may emerge that may be associated with length of stay, care planned, and so forth. The majority of the activities relate to universal self-care adjusted for a health deviation. Health deviation self-care knowledge and performance in managing the condition and its treatment in a broad sense are also listed. As with the nursing diagnosis form, the number of activities according to the level of dependency can be compared between admission and discharge. Further analysis would reveal which activities show

TABLE 8.2 Self-Care Deficit Nursing Theory Outcome Categories

PATIENT
1. Self-care/self-management system
   1.1. Adequate or taking action to modify
   1.2. Integrated into broader system of living
2. Therapeutic self-care demand (actions to meet self-care requisites)
   2.1. Calculates:
      2.1.1. what needs to be done
      2.1.2. how—best method(s) to use
      2.1.3. time sequence
      2.1.4. equipment
   2.2. Adjusts as necessary
   2.3. Actions performed
      2.3.1. quantitatively—complete or not
      2.3.2. qualitatively—how well, consistency
3. Self-care agency
   3.1. General self-care agency
      3.1.1. developed
      3.1.2. exercised
      3.1.3. adequate
   3.2. Self-care operations performed
      3.2.1. knowing
      3.2.2. decision making
      3.2.3. acting
   3.3. Power components
4. Dependent care system
   4.1. In place
   4.2. Adequate or acting to modify
      4.2.1. dependent care operations performed
         4.2.1.1. knowing
         4.2.1.2. decision making
         4.2.1.3. acting
      4.2.2. development of dependent care agency
   4.3. Dependent care system integrated with self-care system of dependent
   4.4. Dependent care system and self-care system of dependent integrated into daily living
   4.5. Dependent care system and self-care system of caregiver(s) integrated into daily living
   4.6. Cooperation and coordination between caregivers if more than one
5. Basic conditioning factors
   5.1. Environment—conditions of living—managing/modifying
   5.2. Health state/system factors—managing
   5.3. Family system factors—managing/modifying
   5.4. Personal sociocultural factors—managing/modifying

TABLE 8.2 *Continued*

NURSING
6. Nursing system
  6.1. Identified self-care limitations
  6.2. Self-care deficits overcome, compensated for
  6.3. Self-care agency maintained, protected
  6.4. Self-care agency increased
  6.5. Dependent care system established, operable, adequate
7. Regulating/monitoring basic conditioning factors
  7.1. Condition, prevention of complications
  7.2. Therapy, effects, results
  7.3. Bodily functions, elimination, etc.
  7.4. Safe, protective use of equipment
  7.5. Safe, protective, supportive physical, social, psychological environment
  7.6. Coordination of communication with other health care services
  7.7. Availability, adequacy of follow-up services

SOURCE: Allison and Renpenning (1998).

the most change and which the least. These data can be examined in relation to basic conditioning factors, type of disability, age, and so on in relation to the power components or self-care operations. They also can be a basis for research to examine the care process and the factors affecting patient outcome.

Theory-Based Patient Classification System

Patient classification systems are management tools. They have been developed primarily as a means for controlling patient care costs in relation to utilization of nursing personnel. However, depending on how they are developed, classification systems also can serve as an outcome measure for evaluating change or maintenance (protection from deterioration) in patient status. Although Pierce (1997) indicated that this had not been documented in the literature, Allison (1989, 1990) presented papers describing the use of a patient classification system for this purpose (see Appendix 8C of this chapter).

Most patient classification systems focus on nursing actions generated by medical orders—medications, treatments, observations of health state and behavior, and routine personal hygienic care provided. All suggest some degree of patient dependency associated with acuity and instability of health condition.

Few define the characteristics of the particular patient population in terms of the reasons that persons are dependent—their self-care limitations and capabilities. If such a system is developed, it can be used as an additional tool for measuring nursing outcomes.

The patient classification system presented in Appendix 8B is based on dependency in self-care of a rehabilitation patient population (Allison, 1988). This system was found to have face and content validity and an inter-rater reliability of 90%. A small correlation study compared it to the Canadian PRN 80 form, which measures the amount of nursing time required to carry out nursing actions to meet neurological patients' needs during a 24-hour period. Tucker (1991) found that a relationship existed between the theoretically based Patient Dependency Scale and the Canadian Nursing Workload Scale.

In the self-care dependency classification system in Appendix 8C, five levels are defined. A zero means that the person is independent and periodically may need reevaluation. It rarely is used for a hospitalized patient unless at the point of discharge. The five levels of dependency range from 1 (*minimally dependent*) to 4 (*completely dependent*) to a fifth category level that encompasses Level 4 but takes into account acuity and instability of the patient that demand close monitoring and care by a registered nurse. Otherwise, what types of nursing personnel are required for the care of these patients is a matter of nursing management judgment based on knowledge of the patients. In rehabilitation, some patients may be totally physically dependent in many aspects of care but physically stable and knowledgeable about their own care. Thus, they should be able to direct the care activities being performed by nursing assistants or other caregivers.

Although this tool gives an estimate of nursing hours, changes in patient status—improvement to a lower level (meaning greater independence) or main-tenance of a desired level—are nursing outcomes. Although some patients—quadriplegics, for example—may never be rated lower than a 3 because of their physical limitations, they may have a great deal of knowledge, will, and reliability in directing others in their care. The tool addresses capabilities and limitations in self-care, showing why nursing assistance is needed, the percent-age in extent of self-care deficits, and stability or instability in health status. The focus of the scale is on physical movement in space and controlled manipulation, as described by Orem (1995) for the basic typology of nursing systems: wholly compensatory, partly compensatory, and supportive-educative (developmental). Such a system needs further refinement. It is an example of another way to measure patient outcomes. This type of tool most frequently is used as a management staffing tool.

Taylor (1990) developed a 12-variable patient classification system for acute medical surgical patients. Each variable is rated on five levels according to the person's capability to manage the element of concern. The 12 variables are (a) lifestyle and family, (b) control of position (mobility), (c) learning and motivation, (d) physiological stability, (e) reaction to illness, (f) behavior, (g) medications and intravenous therapy, (h) feeding and oral fluids, (i) hygiene (personal hygiene and elimination), (j) treatments, (k) infection control, and (l) teaching (amount of information required, language capability). This tool, designed for computerization, has had some testing, but a corresponding workload index has not been developed. An example of the variable of lifestyle and family can be found in Appendix 8C.

Summary

In this chapter, types of patient and nursing outcomes have been examined. The concern of the health care system is whether individuals can manage their health care safely and effectively to promote and maintain their life, health, and well-being and to prevent or reduce use of expensive health care services and facilities. Nursing contributes to these goals by enhancing persons' capabilities to manage their own health care through finding safe, effective, and economical ways to compensate for their lack. Nursing outcomes are identified in terms of persons' self/dependent care capabilities and actions and regulation of factors affecting both. Use of nursing services and/or dependent caregivers also must focus on reducing the need for expensive health care services.

A list of outcome categories based on the self-care deficit theory of nursing is proposed. Examples of types of nursing outcomes are given. A model showing the interdisciplinary perspective on nursing outcomes is presented. The next chapter looks at standards for nursing practice processes to achieve these outcomes, which are based on the self-care deficit nursing theory.

References

Alexander, M. K., Bourgeois, A., & Goodman, L. R. (1994). Total quality improvement: Bridging the gap between education and service. In O. L. Strickland & D. J. Fishman (Eds.), *Nursing issues in the 1990s*. Albany, NY: Delmar.

Allison, S. E. (1988). *Patient classification system*. Unpublished document, Mississippi Methodist Hospital and Rehabilitation Center, Jackson, MS.

Allison, S. E. (1989, October). *Patient outcomes identified through theory-based practice*. Paper presented at the First International Self-Care Deficit Nursing Theory Conference, Kansas City, MO.

Allison, S. E. (1990, September). *Production of nursing outcomes based on Dorothea Orem's self-care deficit nursing theory of nursing.* Paper presented at the National Nursing Theory Conference, University of California at Los Angeles Neuropsychiatric Institute and Hospital Nursing Department, Los Angeles.

American Nurses Association. (1995). *An emerging framework: Data analysis for clinical nursing practice.* Washington, DC: Author.

Association of Operating Room Nurses. (1996). *JCAHO education standards: From challenge to implementation. Patient education, family education, staff education.* Denver, CO: Author.

Avis, M. (1994). Choice cuts: An exploratory study of patients' views about participation in decision-making in a day care surgery unit. *International Journal of Nursing Studies, 31,* 288-298.

Blegen, M. A., Goode, C. J., & Reed, L. (1998). Nurse staffing and patient outcomes. *Nursing Research, 47*(1), 43-50.

Brett, J. L. (1989). Outcome indicators of quality care. In B. Henry, C. Arndt, & M. Di Vincenti (Eds.), *Dimensions of nursing administration* (pp. 362-364). Boston: Blackwell.

Brook, R. H., McGlynn, E. S., & Cleary, P. D. (1996). Quality of health care: Part 2, Measuring quality of care. *New England Journal of Medicine, 34,* 966-970.

Canavan, K. (1996). ANA asserts attacks on practice threaten patient safety. *American Nurse, 28*(1), 1, 9.

Carter, K. F., & Kulbok, P. A. (1995). Evaluation of the interaction model of client health behavior through the first decade of research. *Advances in Nursing Science, 18*(1), 62-73.

Daubert, E. A. (1979). Patient classification system and outcome criteria. *Nursing Outlook, 27,* 450-454.

Donabedian, A. (1968). Evaluating the quality of medical care. *Milbank Memorial Fund Quarterly, 61,* 181-202.

Doswell, W. (1989). The process of measuring patient outcomes. *Journal of New York State Nurses Association, 20*(3), 20-21.

Edwardson, S. R. (1988). Revision and testing of the Hausman and Hegyvary outcome measure for myocardial infarction. In C. F. Waltz & O. L. Strickland (Eds.), *Measurement of nursing outcomes: Vol. 1. Measuring client outcomes* (pp. 24-37). New York: Springer.

Gallant, B. W., & McLane, A. M. (1979). Outcome criteria: A process for validation at the unit level. *Journal of Nursing Administration, 9*(1), 14-20.

Gillis, A. (1995). Exploring nursing outcomes for health promotion. *Nursing Forum, 30*(2), 5-12.

Grohn, M. E., Myers, J., & McSweeney, M. (1996). A comparison of patient acuity and nursing resources in use. *Journal of Nursing Administration, 16*(6), 19-23.

Holzemer, W. (1992, April). *Nursing effectiveness research and patient outcomes.* Paper presented at the Postdoctoral Clinical Seminar of the Western Society for Research in Nursing, San Diego.

Horn, B. J., & Swain, M. A. (1977). *Development of criterion measures of nursing care* (Vols. 1 & 2). Hyattsville, MD: U.S. Department of Commerce, National Technical Information Services.

Kitson, A. L. (1986). Indicators of quality nursing care: An alternate approach. *Journal of Advanced Nursing, 11,* 133-144.

Lee, J. L., & Dean, H. (1995). Patient-education synergy: A research focus on continuity of care. *Nursing Outlook, 43,* 124-126.

Maas, M. L., Johnson, M., & Moorhead, S. (1996). Classifying nursing-sensitive patient outcomes. *Image: Journal of Nursing Scholarship, 28,* 295-301.

Marek, K. D. (1989a). Classification of outcome measures in nursing care. In American Nurses Association (Ed.), *Classification systems for describing nursing practice: Working papers* (pp. 37-42). Washington, DC: American Nurses Association.

Marek, K. D. (1989b). Outcome measurement in nursing. *Journal Nursing Quality Assurance, 4*(11), 1-9.

Meisenheimer, C. G. (1997). *Improving quality: A guide to effective programs.* Gaithersburg, MD: Aspen.

Micek, W. T., Berry, L., Gilski, D., Kallenbach, A., Link, D., & Scharer, K. (1996). Patient outcomes: The links between nursing diagnosis and interventions. *Journal of Nursing Administration, 26*(11), 29-35.

Orem, D. E. (1989). Nursing administration: A theoretical approach. In B. Henry, C. Arndt, M. Di Vincenti, & A. Marriner-Tomey (Eds.), *Dimensions of nursing administration.* Boston: Blackwell.

Orem, D. E. (1990). A nursing theory in three parts, 1956-1989. In M. E. Parker (Ed.), *Nursing theories in practice* (pp. 47-60). New York: National League for Nursing.

Orem, D. E. (1995). *Nursing: Concepts of practice* (5th ed.). St. Louis, MO: Mosby Year-Book.

Pierce, S. F. (1997). Nurse-sensitive health care outcomes in acute care settings: An integrative analysis of the literature. *Journal of Nursing Quality Care, 11*(4), 60-72.

Taylor, S. T. (1990). *Patient classification system.* Unpublished document.

Tucker, D. E. (1991). *The relationship among dependency in self-care, age, and nursing workload of neurological rehabilitation patients.* Unpublished master's thesis, University of Toronto.

Webster's new collegiate dictionary (6th ed.). (1953). Springfield, MA: G. & C. Merriam.

Wunderlich, G. S., Sloan, F. A., & Davis, C. K. (1996). *Nursing staff in hospitals and nursing homes: Is it adequate?* Washington, DC: Institute of Medicine, Division of Health Care Services.

Zander, K. (Ed.). (1995). *Managing outcomes through collaborative case management.* Chicago: American Hospital Association.

Responses About Rehabilitation Outcomes Organized From the Self-Care Deficit Nursing Theory Perspective

In 1996, a group of 10 rehabilitation nurse managers and nurse case managers/clinicians were interviewed to identify what they perceived short- and long-term patient (and particularly nursing) outcomes to be following the patients' discharge from the rehabilitation hospital and over the long term. Using concepts from the self-care deficit nursing theory, a content analysis was done on the verbal responses given. The responses were not tape recorded but were written down briefly. Consequently, it is difficult to determine precisely whether the statement referred to an ability and/or an action.

Not all of the components of the theory were addressed. Those mentioned referred to self-care agency—self-care operations and power components—and to basic conditioning factors, primarily health state and the health care system. Meeting therapeutic self-care demand was implied but not always stated. The outcomes specifically cited as nursing are denoted by a bolded (**N**) after the item.

Self/Dependent Care Agency

1. Self-Care Operations—Productive

  1.1. On discharge

    1.1.1. Productive

      1.1.1.1. Universals adjusted for health deviation

          a. Management of bowel, bladder, and skin (**N**)

          b. Regaining of functional status—dressing, grooming, bed mobility, transfers, bathing, toileting, extended activities of daily living, self-care

          c. Follow-through on things taught in therapies (**N**)

          d. Operation of assistive devices

          e. Making proper arrangements to be in as safe an environment as possible for patient needs

      1.1.1.2. Health deviation self-care

          a. Compliance with medications (**N**)

          b. Adequate pain management (**N**)

    1.1.2. Estimative/transitional

      1.1.2.1. Safety issues related to impulsiveness and to decreased vision, mobility, judgment, and planning abilities (**N**)

      1.1.2.2. Movement in space

      1.1.2.3. Ability to sit in chair for at least 3 to 4 hours and participate in therapy

  1.2. Long range

    1.2.1. Self-care operations—productive

      1.2.1.1. Universals adjusted for health deviation

          a. Effective management of bowel, bladder, and skin care; maintenance of function, prevention of problems (**N**)

          b. Increased mobility

    c. Maintenance of appropriate weight and safety, intake of food and fluids, skin integrity and precautions (N)

    d. Seeking assistance as needed

    e. Catheterization every 6 to 7 hours without reservoir leaking

    f. Patient/family's ability to manage their care needs effectively (N)

1.2.1.2. Developmental self-care (mentioned as such)

    a. Maintenance of as much independence as physically/mentally possible

    b. Being socially functional, returning to daily activities, school, work, etc. (N)

1.2.1.3. Health deviation self-care (mentioned as such)

    a. Compliance with/management of medications, adjusting with diet (swallowing program)

2. Power Components

2.1. On discharge

2.1.1. Technical knowledge

2.1.1.1. Universals

    a. Demonstrated understanding of home care through discussion and return demonstration

    b. Ability to manage bowel, bladder, and skin programs

2.1.2. Health deviation self-care

2.1.2.1. Knowledge base enhancement concerning medications, stroke extension precautions, safe and adequate nutritional intake, management of urinary diversion and expected outcomes, anticoagulant treatment, preventive measures for risk factors and warning signs related to illness/medications, needs for supplies and how to receive assistance from organizations, coordination of home care, wound care/treatment, home services (N)

2.1.3. Dependent care agency

2.1.3.1. Caregiver adequate knowledge and understanding of home care services

2.2. Long range

2.2.1. Caregiver knowledge and understanding of home program and management

Basic Conditioning Factors

1. On discharge

1.1. Health state

1.1.1. Adequate bowel and bladder function, free of or adequate healing of skin breakdown

1.2. Health system factors

1.2.1. Follow-up care arrangements—home health, clinic

1.2.2. Patient has proper equipment

1.2.3. Education of patient/primary caregiver been completed (**N**)

1.2.4. Providing efficient therapy/cutting costs

1.2.5. Discharge goals are met

2. Long range

2.1. Health state

2.1.1. Decrease/absence of complications—blood clots, urinary tract infections, other infections that affect readmissions, constipation

Nursing Agency

1. On discharge

1.1. Patient/family education has been completed (**N**)

1.2. Equipment (nursing) available

1.3. Appropriate follow-up

1.4. Coordination of services

Insurance Company Concerns Expressed

---

1. Self-care agency—self-care operations—productive
    1.1. Families know about home care and follow-up
    1.2. Return to work, school, community
2. Basic conditioning factors
    2.1. Health state—medically stable
    2.2. Health care system—prevent readmissions due to secondary complications, early interventions concerning problems management, home care needs met, have needed equipment, team recommendations are appropriate to patients' needs, adequate follow-up; cost containment—placement appropriate, length of stay decreased, vendor selections (re: costs), early intervention (re: problems), prevention of readmissions

Reasons Why a Home Visit Is Needed on Discharge

When the nurses were asked why every patient should have a home visit following hospital discharge, the reasons given, in a sense, were outcomes. They included

1. Check safety
2. Check that equipment is in place as needed
3. Check compliance with home care—medication, follow-through
4. Continue service through coordination with home health nurse
5. Assess medical problems
6. See patients who cannot be contacted via telephone follow-up calls (can reach only 10% now)
7. See if what was planned is happening
8. See how caregiver is managing
9. Was placement decision appropriate?
10. Observe the social/physical environment

Patient Self-Care
Classification

Level	Capabilities	Limitations	Self-Care Deficits	Conditioning Factors	Nursing Assistance Needed
0 INDEPENDENT	PRESENT AND ADEQUATE	NONE	NONE	NONE	NONE: REEVALUATE AS NECESSARY
1 MINIMALLY DEPENDENT	PRESENT AND GENERALLY ADEQUATE	Difficulty remembering, making decisions about some aspects of care	PARTIAL Selected knowledge/ procedures— 20% or less of actions	CONDITION— STABLE Hospital policies limit performance (e.g., medications)	EDUCATE, GUIDE, AND SUPPORT To manage new situation, develop and refine self-care
(Hours care/day less than 1-2)	Has basic knowledge and skills, judgments, and willingness	Variable physical/emotional energy to perform all of care		Special diagnostic/treatments to be performed	
		Uninterested/unwilling to carry out selected procedures at this time		Lacks necessary equipment and supplies	
	Requests assistance as needed	Lacks sufficient knowledge about specific/new health care measures required			
	Performs more than 80% of activities independently				

2 MODERATELY DEPENDENT (Hours of care/day 2.1-3.5)	PRESENT— INCOMPLETE AND INADEQUATE Some basic knowledge; is learning and developing skills in rehab program Performs 50% or more of care independently or with equipment	Knowledge and skills insufficient for new temporary/permanent event May not always make safe decisions, remember or be willing to engage in self-care on a consistent basis Method of communication may be slow/difficult Problems with adjustment to disability affect output of effort or engagement in some activities Tires too easily to complete activities	PARTIAL 50% of care	CONDITION STABLE; MAY BE EXPERIENCING SOME DISCOMFORT New or somewhat stressful event such as surgery, recovery from minor surgery Family/significant other intervenes/prevents engagement in activities Pain limits activities	As above, plus help with activities of daily living and to complete care and transportation: for example, may be mobile in wheelchair/gurney but require transfer assistance and aid with special treatments Requires teaching, guiding, supervision with the above, emotional support, developmental environment to maximize function, engage in activities, go through procedures and therapy

Level	Capabilities	Limitations	Self-Care Deficits	Conditioning Factors	Nursing Assistance Needs
3 HEAVILY DEPENDENT (Hours of care/day 3.6-6)	PARTIALLY PRESENT, INADEQUATE Usually aware with beginning knowledge about disability and rehab program Cooperates as able Performs 20% of care activities	General lack of knowledge about what and how to do; or may be knowledgeable and experienced but physically temporarily unable to manage without usual lay caregiver Cognitive impairment limits learning and reasoning about self-care May be mobile but gets lost if unescorted Severe emotional adjustment to disability; immaturity or other factors inhibit performance or willingness to engage in rehab program: e.g., denial, difficult to satisfy making numerous minor requests Physical inability to move due to extent of disability or newness of injury or impairment Excessive slowness	PARTIAL Up to 80% of activities	CONDITION: STABLE Cognitive deficits: limited intelligence, short attention span, confusion, forgetfulness, impairment in judgment and decision-making abilities Communication impairment Depression/anxiety Medical condition/treatment imposes physical limitations, requires special observations and care (e.g., elderly "fresh" stroke patient, recent postoperative patient, spinal cord injury patient "just getting up," pain management) Medical prescription limits activity Experienced highly disabled rehab patient without caregiver admitted for medical complication	Physical assistance required for 80% of care— grooming, dressing, feeding, transfers, transportation Intensive education and support, development of environment to promote initiation and carry through in rehab program Family support and education on therapeutic regime and disability

4 COMPLETELY DEPENDENT	PRESENT, PARTIALLY DEPENDENT, OPERABLE TO INOPERABLE, INADEQUATE	CANNOT OR SHOULD NOT ATTEMPT TO PERFORM MOST OF PHYSICAL ACTIVITIES	COMPLETE	CONDITION: At risk of instability; acute illness episode or severity of impairment re: cognitive, emotional, and/or medical modalities used: e.g., tracheotomy, ventilator, monitoring	Frequent, at least once-an-hour monitoring and care from a licensed nurse over an extended 24-hour period re: cardiorespiratory and neurological status
24-hour period (hours care/day 6.1-8)	May be aware, able to communicate	Not alert or physically able, knowledgeable to monitor self/treatment	90% of activities or more	Anxious family	Protection from hazards and complications
	Cooperates to extent able				Provision of guidance and support to patient and family members (RN direct care or close RN supervision of LPN)
	May perform 10% of self-care activities				

Level	Capabilities	Limitations	Self-Care Deficits	Conditioning Factors	Nursing Assistance Needs
5 TOTALLY DEPENDENT, ACUTELY ILL	INOPERABLE/ INADEQUATE	MINIMAL TO NO ABILITY TO EXPRESS NEEDS, WISHES	COMPLETE	CONDITION: UNSTABLE	CONSTANT MONITORING AND CARE BY A REGISTERED NURSE (Constant Care Unit)
(Hours care/day 8 and above)	Partial awareness Possible limited ability to communicate	Physically, mentally, emotionally limited in volitional functioning	About 100%	Undergoing frequent change in condition requires close supervision and treatment regarding invasive monitoring, control and electrolytes, cardiopulmonary status and function	Management of cardiac, respiratory, fluid, medication support systems
				UNCONTROLLED, UNCONTROLLED and DETERIORATING	Family support
				Distressed family	

Excerpt From a Classification System Developed in an Acute Care Setting

LIFESTYLE AND FAMILY

1. The patient has a history of having been responsible for his/her own care, having coped successfully with stress situations, and/or having a positive attitude toward his/her health. There is a positive family social support. Sexuality needs are met. Family demonstrates ability to cope with patient illness.

2. Patient has slight difficulty in coping with illness. Individual lifestyle impacts on ability to care for self. Family requires minimal assistance and/or support in coping with the patient's illness.

3. Patient is limited in his/her ability to care for self due to pain, preoccupation, or stress of illness. There is impairment of sexual satisfaction. Lifestyle, including work and family and outside demands, is causing stress. Family requires assistance in gaining knowledge of how to support patient. Family has ability to cope with patient illness but requires moderate support.

AUTHORS' NOTE: Used with permission of Dr. Susan Taylor.

4. The patient has extensive difficulty in caring for self due to age, individual lifestyle, culture or inability to cope with the stress of illness. Inability to meet sexuality needs causing significant stress. Patient has no family or significant other or family places extensive demands on staff for support and assistance.

5. Patient is unable to care for self due to age, individual lifestyle, culture, or the inability to cope with the stress of illness. Family is unable to cope with patient illness and requires maximum support.

Comments:

Quality Control

Nursing Standards

S tandards are the basis for evaluating nursing. They are both the goals to be achieved and the guides for conduct. Nursing standards comprise (a) *standards of practice,* which focus on what nurses should do and how they should do it; and (b) *standards of care,* which focus on what patients/clients should receive—the product of nursing. In this chapter, the focus is on how the self-care deficit nursing theory provides direction for specifying some of the standards of practice and helps to delineate standards of care. Examples of both kinds of standards are presented.

Standards of Practice

Standards of practice are incorporated into legislation governing the practice of nursing. Professional associations and clinical practice specialties publish standards of practice. Standards of practice are developed within the guidelines of the legal authority for the practice of the profession within the health care enterprise. All of these standards are discussed in non-discipline-specific terms. This discussion will be confined to how a nursing practice theory influences the content of the standards, facilitating the development of criterion indicators that the standards are being met and the development of tools for measuring outcomes.

Nursing standards of practice focus on what nurses should do and how they should do it: that is, what should be done at certain times and how to accomplish certain goals. For example, a nursing assessment must be done within a specified time of admission to a service to determine what needs to be done for the patient and to establish nursing goals and a nursing prognosis. Nursing procedures are standards for performing certain techniques, and protocols are standard guidelines for determining what actions to perform or not perform and when to perform them.

Standards of practice within an organization should be consistent with the overall philosophy and mission of the enterprise. They should be consistent with the mental model espoused by the practitioners. If self-care deficit nursing theory is accepted as the framework for practice in an organization, then as a standard of practice all nurses will be expected to focus on the self-care systems of the patients/clients. Nurses will attend to the relationships among conditioning factors, self-care demand, and self-care capabilities. They will design nursing systems that focus on the social, interpersonal, and technological aspects of care as appropriate to the period of time in which they are involved with the patient, including planning for continuity of care over time where appropriate.

Written protocols and procedures also can reflect direction from self-care deficit nursing theory. For example, in writing a protocol or procedure related to isolation, in addition to all of the "things" that must be attended to, attention should be directed to particular aspects of the self-care demand that might be affected by the procedure, such as promotion of development, promotion of normalcy, maintenance of a sufficient intake of food, and maintenance of a balance between rest and activity.

The performance appraisal system is the tool for evaluating the extent to which the nurses meet the standards of practice. Criteria for the performance appraisal might include evidence that the nurses are attending to self-care, are designing appropriate nursing systems, and are evaluating the capability of family members to perform aspects of the required care.

Standards of Care

Standards of care focus on what patients/clients should receive: that is, both the quality and the quantity of care. The evidence that standards of care have been met is reflected in patient variables. Without a theory base to identify those variables, the measures used are often evaluations of patient satisfaction or standards and outcome measures related to progress regarding medical therapies. Only in recent years, through delineation of clinical paths, have nurses begun to establish standards of care from a process perspective. Zander (1995), in collaboration with medical staff, led the way and continues this work. The nursing activities in Zander's standards include monitoring, administration of medications and treatments, and patient teaching. The role and activities of the patient in these clinical paths tend to be implicit, not explicit. The role and functions delineated for the nurse may be limited to routine nursing procedures and monitoring of health status and response to treatments. There is little or no reference to determining the extent of development of appropriate self-care management systems or to development, adequacy, and operability of self-care agency as goals to be attained. Table 9.1 shows a care map incorporating concepts from self-care deficit nursing theory.

Self-care deficit nursing theory provides a means of looking at the whole scope of nursing care required by the patient, thereby facilitating specification of the content for the standards of care reflective of the domain of nursing. For example, when a nurse assesses a patient, the theory provides a systematic approach not unlike that of medicine. When a physician does a history and physical, the standard medical examination proceeds from "head to toe." When a nurse uses self-care deficit nursing theory, the self-care requisites—universal, developmental, health deviation—are systematically investigated and related to the basic conditioning factors or ruled out as is pertinent to the situation. Similarly, types of actions to meet the requisites are determined in light of the person's self-care abilities and limitations influencing them. Examination of the theory variables in terms of patient populations thus becomes a standard of care (Department of Nursing, 1990).

When self-care deficit nursing theory is used to guide the development of standards of care, the standards address what the patient should be expected to know and do at particular stages of care and the desired results at the end of each stage. They include what the patient or family member should or should not be able to do at particular points in time. In addition, there are standards related to provision of care to meet the self-care demand and to protect or develop self-care/dependent care agency. Evaluation criteria include the extent to which and circumstances under which the self-care demand is or is not met and goals related to self-care/dependent care agency are accomplished.

When working from the self-care deficit nursing theory perspective, then, consideration can be given to identification of

TABLE 9.1 Design of a Care Map Integrating Variables From Self-Care Deficit Nursing Theory

Focus of Concern	Day 1	Day 2	Day 3	Day 4	Day 5
Maintenance of sufficient intake of air	Explanations Suctioning Monitor vital signs rate q 15 min for 1 hour postop., then q4h for 24 hrs	Reassure Deep breathing and coughing with assistance Vital signs q4h Hgb	Support Deep breathing and coughing independent Monitor pulmonary sounds	Encourage pt. to continue with deep breathing and coughing if necessary	Pt. initiates deep breathing and coughing on own
Maintenance of sufficient intake of water	NPO IV as ordered	Fluids as tolerated with IV supplement up to __ ml	1,500 ml per day Evaluate understanding of fluid requirements Instruct prn	Pt. monitors own fluid intake	
Balance of rest and activity	Bed rest Describe what to expect regarding ambulation	In chair x2 with assistance Involve pt. in ambulation	Bathroom privileges Teach about energy saving Incorporate feedback from patient	Up ad lib Pt. incorporates energy saving Involve family Incorporate feedback from family	Pt./family demonstrate and verbalize strategies for balancing rest/activity at home
Care regarding elimination	Monitor indwelling catheter Measure output q8h	Monitor catheter Measure output q8h	Remove catheter Measure residual	Monitor output Observe for retention	
Motivation—confidence to care for self	Explain what is happening Reassure as to normalcy of course of events	Continue to explain, reassure, involve in activity depending on physical state/energy	Support efforts to participate	Pt./family should be doing most things	Pt./family should be able to manage required care

1. The outcome indicators listed
2. Therapeutic self-care demand
3. Exercise of self-care agency in patient actions
4. Nursing actions in relation to patient actions
5. The outcome thresholds desired

Indicators may be established for selected intervals of care, as in a care map. As mentioned in the previous chapter, outcomes generally are interpreted as measurable change but also may be stated in terms of maintaining or protecting an action or a capability for action. Obviously, also, outcomes in terms of general health goals—for example, control of diabetes, prevention of complications, and reduction of hospital length of stay—are parameters to be measured. But achievement of these goals should be related to self/dependent care status: the effectiveness, adequacy, and consistency in exercise of actions through estimative, transitional, and productive self-care operations. These can be reflected in the standards.

Examples From the Clinical Arena

In practice, it is very difficult to separate standards of practice and standards of care because they are interrelated. This section presents two examples of nursing standards reflective of both practice and care that have been framed from the perspective of self-care deficit nursing theory.

A Bowel Management Standard

The format for nursing standards will vary by institution or agency. Many examples can be found in the literature. In the rehabilitation hospital whose philosophy is presented in Chapter 5, the standards were set up on the basis of the Joint Commission for Accreditation of Health Care Organizations format in the 1980s. A set of nursing standards for a bowel management program is presented in Appendix 9A (Spinal Cord Injury Service, 1990). Four areas are addressed in the standards: outcome indicators, nursing actions, patient actions, and outcome thresholds.

The standards specifically address activities involved in a bowel management program for persons with paralysis from spinal cord injury. They also apply to those with brain injury whose bowel elimination is affected at a different level. Three indicators used are

1. Identification of the bowel status (normalcy/abnormalcy) on admission to the facility
2. Regulation of elimination and effectiveness of current treatment measures
3. Ability/limitations of patient/caregiver to manage the elimination process

Thresholds for achievement of these goals are stated. The thresholds can be revised up or down after evaluation of results and processes over a period of time.

Example From Community Health

Another system of nursing assessment standards based on the self-care deficit nursing theory, illustrated in Appendix 9B, is the extensive work done by the nurses of the Vancouver Health Department (1988). Because Vancouver is a multicultural city, cultural factors are taken into account in the development of these nursing standards. Relevant differences, particularly around child care, are addressed. The category items analyzed are

1. Actions to be taken by the client (self-care demand)
2. Knowledge, skill, ability to take action (self-care agency)
3. Sociocultural factors influencing them
4. Nursing actions

These standards serve as an assessment tool, a practice process standard, and a standard care plan that includes dates of initiation, progress, and completion.

Similarly, the standards for the rehabilitation patient population can serve as standard care plans aiding nursing documentation. One caution about standardization is the need to keep an open mind to discern individual differences. Observe and listen to patients and their caregivers so as not to exclude important information or concerns expressed. Each individual presents a unique situation, and nurses must flexibly adjust and attend to these variations. Measurement of achievement of the standards and outcomes, of course, depends on the adequacy and consistency of nursing documentation and observations of the performance of nursing personnel.

TABLE 9.2 Framework to Establish Standards of Care for a Patient or Category of Patients

GOALS

To maintain good health or to develop better health, the patient/dependent care agent must know and/or do: (Identify/specify)

To carry out the prescribed plan of therapy to correct or limit the health condition, the patient/dependent care agent must know and/or do: (Identify/specify)

THE HEALTH CARE ACTION

What will be done by the patient/dependent care agent

Which assistances will be needed to make the action meet acceptable standards

THE ROLES OF NURSING IN THESE HEALTH ACTIONS

CAPACITIES

Patient/dependent care capacities that affect doing these actions:

Capabilities

Limitations

EFFECT OF THE SITUATION

Effect of the situation in which care is given on the patient's actions

SOURCE: Backscheider (1970).

A Framework for Establishing Nursing Standards

A general framework for establishing nursing standards of care for a patient or a category of patients is shown in Table 9.2.

The central focus of this framework is on the health care actions to be taken by the patient/client and the assistances (nursing) needed to make each action meet acceptable standards: for example, all the necessary steps in insulin administration. These actions are taken in light of two main goals: The first is management of the prescribed therapies for a particular health condition, and the second is maintenance or development of health and well-being in general. Factors to be addressed affecting the health care actions are the capabilities and limitations of the patient/dependent care agent related to carrying out the actions and the effects of the situation—home, hospital, and other factors—on the patient's or dependent care agent's actions. The role of nursing in relation to these required health (self-care) actions can be delineated. This framework simply shows what to think about in setting up the standard; the particular approach in setting up standards will vary with the institution or agency and the philosophy of nursing.

The standards described earlier for bowel management for the spinal cord injury patient (Appendix 9A) list some general nursing actions. The selected example does not specifically address patient capabilities per se except in terms of types of limitations that may preclude or alter meeting these general standards; nor does it address general health goals. This would require a separate standard.

Summary

Standards of practice are concerned with what nurses should do and how to do it. In this chapter, the contribution of the self-care deficit nursing theory in providing direction for a systematic approach to development of standards is discussed. The theory provides a framework for specifying a standard of care in that it helps to determine what persons are doing, should do, and can do in managing their own health care. In the case of caregivers (dependent care agents), the theory guides exploration into how they are managing in light of their own capabilities, activities, desires, and the situation in relation to appropriate courses of action. Use of self-care deficit nursing is one way to ensure that nursing standards relating to both practice and care truly focus on the patient/client.

References

Backscheider, J. E. (1970). *Working papers*. Unpublished documents, Woman's Clinic Project, Center for Experimentation and Development in Nursing, Johns Hopkins Hospital, Baltimore.

Department of Nursing, Mississippi Methodist Hospital and Rehabilitation Center. (1990). *Standards of care*. Unpublished document, Jackson, MS.

Spinal Cord Injury Service, Mississippi Methodist Hospital and Rehabilitation Center. (1990). *Nursing standards for bowel management*. Unpublished document, Jackson, MS.

Vancouver Health Department. (1988) *Assessment standards*. Vancouver, Canada: Author.

Zander, K. (Ed.). (1995) *Managing outcomes through collaborative case management*. Chicago: American Hospital Association.

Excerpt From Nursing Standards for Bowel Management for Patients With Spinal Cord Injury

AUTHORS' NOTE: These nursing standards are those of the Spinal Cord Injury Service of the Mississippi Methodist Hospital and Rehabilitation Center, Jackson, MS (1990; revised 1998). Reprinted courtesy of the Department of Nursing of the Mississippi Methodist Hospital and Rehabilitation Center.

2A. OUTCOME STANDARD

Each patient's bowel function (normal/abnormal) will be regulated with a bowel program to meet the individual's needs by the time of hospital discharge.

2B. PROCESS STANDARD

An individualized bowel program will be established and maintained for patients whose normal bowel function is disrupted by conditions/treatments.

2C. OUTCOME	NURSING ACTIONS	PATIENT ACTION
By discharge the patient or dependent care agent will demonstrate ability to plan, manage, and regulate a bowel program identified by individual goals in the patient's care plan.	RN will: 1. Assess with the patient/family capabilities and limitations in management of the bowel program. 2. Identify individual specific learning goals with the patient or family. 3. Design and implement an individual bowel program with the patient and family using resource persons, established learning programs, and approved nursing procedures associated with bowel function management. Refer to Spinal Injury Learning Series, Bowel Management Education Progress Note, and Nursing Procedures. 4. Document evaluation of progress in learned bowel progress and discharge notes.	1. Patient or family will provide information. 2. Patient and/or family will cooperate in identifying goals. 3. Patient and or family will listen to and demonstrate ability to perform parts of the program as follows: 3.1. Verbalize and demonstrate knowledge of high-fiber diet or fluid intake. 3.2. Verbalize/demonstrate transfer to bed/commode chair/toilet. 3.3. Verbalize/demonstrate donning gloves and inserting suppository and cleanup. 3.4. Know name, action, reaction of bowel medications.

EXCEPTIONS TO STANDARDS:

1. Early discharge/transfer
2. Recent ostomy
3. Complicating condition/treatment
4. Refusal of program/lack of readiness
5. Documented evidence of no bowel management problems

OUTCOME	EVALUATION
By discharge 80% of the patient/families will demonstrate achievement of individual program, achievement of individual goals; see nursing care plan.	As documented in the progress note, Bowel Education form, daily Nursing Consult form or Nursing Summary.

Excerpt From Nursing
Assessment Standards

**Population: 0-28 Days Postpartum
(Chinese Maternal Adaptation)**

This clinical population is Chinese women in childbearing years who have a baby aged 0-28 days. This population has a varied background, as the women may have been born in Hong Kong, China, Taiwan, elsewhere in Southeast Asia, or Canada. Cultural practices will vary depending upon their birthplace, educational and socioeconomic background. The extended family, especially the older generation, has a strong influence on the postpartum practices, helps the new mother, and may even take over the care of the baby.

The postpartum practices are rooted in the Chinese theory of health, which is based on the balance of Yin and Yang. Yin is female, negative, and cool, while Yang is male, positive, and hot. After the baby's birth, the woman's body is considered to have an excess of Yin, so more Yang foods are eaten to achieve a balance. Also, the woman is considered to be susceptible to "wind" or *feng,* which is a noxious substance that can enter the body and cause illness. To avoid this the woman stays indoors for one month and limits contact with water. The

AUTHORS' NOTE: The materials in this appendix come from unpublished documents of the Vancouver Health Department, Vancouver, Canada. Materials reprinted courtesy of the Vancouver/ Richmond Health Board.

guide reflects the strictest practices that traditional Chinese women may follow. Generally, the postpartum restrictions are dietary, so Yin foods are avoided, and more Yang foods, especially ginger, are eaten.

The self-care and dependent care agency of the Chinese women are usually well developed. The birth of a baby is an important event. Doctors and nurses are viewed with respect, and the doctor is the ultimate authority. Conflicts may occur if the nurse's advice differs from the doctor's.

Results Sought Through Nursing Actions

- Promoting optimal maternal and infant health
- Observing and respecting cultural beliefs and practices
- Increasing knowledge and understanding of anatomy and physiology of labour and birth (Chinese women usually do not attend prenatal classes)
- Providing information about the potential effects of dietary restrictions on postpartum recovery and breast feeding

Actions to Be Taken by Client (Self-Care Demand)	Knowledge, Skill, Ability to Take Action (Self-Care Agency)	Sociocultural Factors	Nursing Actions
Provides care associated with elimination processes and excrements

Reestablishes normal pattern of bowel elimination by 3-5 days postpartum. Acts to counteract factors contributing to constipation if indicated | Knowledge of normal pattern

Awareness of current pattern

Knowledge of measures to take to reestablish normal pattern

Knowledge of factors contributing to constipation | Most Chinese mothers, if they are constipated, will consult their doctor rather than making dietary changes | Discuss causes of constipation and encourage increasing fluids and fibre in diet |
| Takes appropriate action if lochia abnormal | Vocabulary to describe lochia

Knows who to contact about abnormalities | Openly discuss lochia and perineal care even if husband present | Observe lochia if appropriate |

Fiscal Management and Delivery of Safe, Effective Nursing

The lack of an adequate definition of nursing reflected in most databases is a major impediment to budgeting and costing of nursing services. Nursing theory is useful in helping the nurse administrator to determine nursing costs and allocate resources for delivery of safe, effective nursing. Determining nursing costs is complex and necessary for developing appropriate budgets. Nursing theory can help the administrator meet some of these challenges. As indicated previously, nursing theory provides a basis for specifying the domain and boundaries of nursing and provides direction for development of the clinical information system and for establishing and measuring outcomes. All are foundational to developing ways of costing nursing services, a budget for nursing services, and appropriate fiscal management systems. A significant goal is to demonstrate that nursing can be a revenue generator as well as a revenue consumer.

The Complexity of Costing Nursing Services

Ideally, fiscal management is concerned with utilization of resources at least cost to attain the goals of the health care enterprise and to achieve economic outputs: beneficial patient outcomes, efficiency of operations, and, where applicable, maximization of profits. Economic value is attached to the intensity of resource use—the level and kind of services provided by the nursing service organization to attain desired results. Given the financial concerns about the costs of health care, it is incumbent on nursing to define its costs, benefits, and outputs and to explore improved and innovative approaches for the delivery of safe, effective nursing in a cost-effective manner.

Prospective payment (incentives to control costs) and capitation (allowance of a defined amount of money per individual patient for all health care provided) are realities. Resources for nursing and other health services may be severely limited. Justification of need and evidence of results or benefits attained must be specified to obtain resources. Historically, costing out nursing has been done on the basis of studies of time spent in selected nursing activities. Reliance is placed on the best experiential judgments about use of nursing resources needed to provide nursing for a particular group of patients.

Generally, three methods have been used to cost out nursing: (a) the per diem method, in which costs are related to length of stay; (b) relative intensity measures (RIMs), in which registered nurse (RN) minutes equivalents are derived from salary conversions rather than skill needed; and (c) nursing workload, based on patient acuity and time estimates for nursing activities and the patient classification system to determine the staffing mix needed. Other methods have been tried with varying degrees of success. These include determining units of service by nursing diagnosis, nursing care plans per diagnosis-related group (DRG), and estimates of time and personnel costs based on standards of care. Some of these categorize nursing actions as dependent on physician orders or independent of them (Edwardson & Giovanneti, 1987; Flarey, 1990; Sherman, 1990).

An adequate costing system enables better management assessment and control, better utilization of resources, and greater productivity (Flarey, 1990). Flarey further noted that a detailed costing system for nursing requires an in-depth understanding of nursing as a science as well as knowledge of the nursing and medical needs of patients. Of particular significance is the point that nursing should be viewed as a revenue-producing center and not simply as an expense.

Sherman (1990) cited the need for an objective national system for identifying nursing costs. She noted that a number of variables affect nursing care beyond consideration of patient needs and staff mix. These include the type of delivery system used, the mission and philosophy, the standards of the institution, physician practice patterns, the physical plant, supplies, and support services. Sherman also noted the difficulty of using patient records for retrospective audits because of the lack of documentation of independent nursing functions. She identified a need, for cost accounting purposes, for charges or costs to be assigned to a nursing activity and to direct patient care at the time the service is provided. When documented this way, real nursing costs can be identified daily and throughout a patient's stay or course of service. The lack of documentation of nursing is also frequently cited as an issue in articles dealing with informatics and nursing. Retrospective audits to determine nursing costs are inadequate because of the limitations of current documentation systems (Androwich & Stoupa, 1994; Milholland, 1992) and lack of specification of nursing.

Incorporation of managed-care strategies into delivery systems is currently being promoted as a method to control costs. Clinical paths have become essential tools of the managed-care movement. Articles are appearing in the literature in which attempts are being made to cost out clinical pathways. Gardner, Allhusen, Kamm, and Tobin (1997) proposed two methods for determining cost of care through clinical pathways. Integral to both of these methods is specifying the nursing component and having a clinical information system to provide data about that system. There is no clear indication in the article that the factors influencing nursing productivity as described by Flarey and Sherman are included at this point in the development of the costing formulas.

A Metaparadigm for Studying Nursing Work

Building on a 1993 study (Cockerill, O'Brien-Pallas, Bolley, & Pink, 1993), related work (Cockerill & O'Brien-Pallas, 1990; Halloran, 1985; Jelinek, 1967), and a literature review, the research team of O'Brien-Pallas, Irvine, Peereboom, and Murray (1997) presented a metaparadigm for studying nursing intensity costs. It can help nurse administrators to understand that work and help non-nurse administrators to understand the breadth and scope of nursing and factors influencing productivity. It includes patient nursing complexity, nursing characteristics, environmental complexity, medical condition, and condition severity. The authors' report of a study operationalizing the basic constructs of the metaparadigm (O'Brien-Pallas et al., 1997) suggests that incorporating self-care deficit nursing theory into that paradigm could provide further understanding of nursing work and related costs.

The self-care deficit nursing theory provides structure for identifying both the nursing process elements (elements of the service to be provided) and nursing outcomes (types of results achieved in terms of overcoming actual or potential self-care deficits and addressing the reasons for them) in selected patient populations. These general outcomes can be particularized to individual patients. The types of nursing actions required usually can be generally predicted in clinical care maps for subpopulations and then particularized to individual nursing cases. Nursing resources then can be allocated on the basis of these general designs of nursing systems. Development of designs of nursing systems for patient populations and subpopulations aids in setting standards for nursing care, which can be a basis for costing nursing services. The foundation for approaching costing of nursing from this perspective has been already been laid:

- In Chapter 2's identification of variables of concern to nursing
- In Chapter 3's conceptualization of nursing as an entity across organizational units or as a unit within a larger unit
- In Chapter 4's schema for describing patient populations
- In Chapter 6's model for designing nursing for populations
- In Chapter 7's direction given for including the variables of concern to nursing in the clinical information system and documentation aids
- In Chapter 8's schema for identification of outcome categories
- In Chapter 9's identification of the content related to standards

Chapter 11 will also contribute to this foundation by providing direction for differentiating levels of practice.

Nursing Administration Role

The challenge to nursing administration is to establish reasonable goals for the particular health care situation (agency or institution) and to establish linkages with other health care services to ensure follow-up and continuity of care in collaboration with them. This is a monumental task for nursing administration in this age of cost cutting, but the goal of cost reduction should be to achieve the best results within budgetary constraints and not inadequacies that may ultimately have costly results. In other words, health care benefits should take precedence over cutting bottom-line costs.

Without more definitive means for costing nursing services, continued reimbursement to hospitals and service agencies may be based on room rates, clinic visits, and fees charged for selected services in hospitals, outpatient services, and home health agencies. Nursing budget estimates tend to be based on past experience, shift coverage, and other factors affecting a 24-hour service, such as on-call pay, shift differentials, and overtime. These estimates do not relate use of nursing resources to achievement of particular nursing outcomes for a patient population or subpopulation.

Changing the method for describing and for costing nursing services requires a specification of the nursing focus that enables definition of nursing outcomes and delineation of nursing processes—the nursing systems needed—to achieve them. Clinical care maps are a beginning, but many lack a specific nursing focus outlining nurse and patient actions (outcomes to be achieved) in the health care process. Without this focus, nursing budgets will continue to be based primarily on workload estimates without the concept of productivity in terms of results achieved through nursing effort by different types and levels of nursing workers. Cost cutting to reduce dollars has occurred and will continue in terms of reducing the number and quality of nursing personnel. A recent study reports the negative impact of this on nursing care and quality of patient outcomes (Canavan, 1997). Reduced staffing results in frustration among nurses because of work overload and a lack of the sense of accomplishment and satisfaction that is derived from providing safe, effective nursing care.

Zero-based budgeting—annual justification "from-scratch" estimates of nursing personnel and other needs to provide necessary services—requires sound clinical data and financial data. Justification of resource use in terms of results to be achieved clinically and financially and in terms of revenue generation is essential for appropriate nursing budget projections. This moves nursing out of the expense category into a revenue-generating one, a service contributing to the productivity of the enterprise and possibly enabling or enhancing some profit. Nurse administrators are tested not simply to reduce costs but to be innovative in providing and marketing nursing services and in retaining and developing competent nursing personnel.

Various strategies are being tried. Integration of nursing personnel with other health care services to work as teams, particularly in ambulatory care and home health, is one strategy. Another is to cross-train nurses to work in a variety of health care environments. For example, one community hospital that was experiencing a reduction in patient care days, rather than laying off nurses, sought to promote continuity of nursing care. The nursing department was redesigned, and inpatient nurses were reassigned and taught to provide home health care. That, in turn, promoted nurse and patient satisfaction through follow-up care (Donlevey & Pietruch, 1996). Another organizational approach is decentralization to reduce the number of personnel and management layers to the operational level in the nursing organization (Pinkerton, 1996). The aim here is to bring about greater accountability along with responsibility at the work operations level.

The challenge to nursing administrators and nursing practitioners is to be aware of the economic impact as well as the required care components of their world. This means they must know how to maximize their time, seek work simplification methods, design appropriate and effective ways to utilize nursing personnel, and use electronic communication to facilitate documentation of care and record services rendered for cost accounting as well as clinical purposes. Nursing administration must become adept not only at balancing expenses against revenues to offset costs but at becoming revenue generating. Nurse administrators need to become entrepreneurs as well as innovators to ensure that needed nursing services are made available cost-effectively. For example, this can occur through nurse-conducted clinics using physician consultation as necessary and through collaborative efforts in health care teams between nursing and other health care disciplines. In primary care programs, for instance, nurses should develop strong educative-supportive nursing systems to promote health maintenance and prevention of illness through the clients' enhanced self/dependent care systems.

Budget Model

Nursing administration and advanced practitioners of nursing must design nursing systems for patient populations that identify nursing costs as a basis for setting nursing prices for the services provided and address the factors affecting both. In the model in Figure 10.1, dimensions for budgeting—forecasting, providing for, distributing, and financing nursing—are delineated.

In Table 10.1, the budget elements to be analyzed and projected are delineated for the particular situation. Effective budgeting entails planning for implementation, close collaboration with other health team members, and accurate and timely record keeping—point-of-service documentation and monitoring by participants to ensure control of costs while providing safe, effective care. Depending on the pricing structure of the institution or agency, the price markup

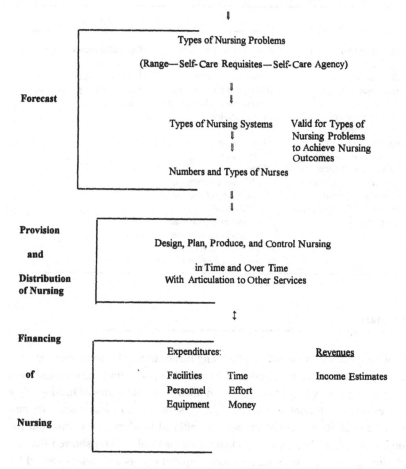

Figure 10.1. Considerations in Nursing Administration

may range from 10% to 100% or more over cost. This is highly variable depending on profit motive and reimbursement allocations.

Essential to all of this is making clear to nurses, the public, and other health care professionals what nursing goals and outcomes are and justifying the resources needed to achieve them. The models presented can be a beginning basis for examining and costing out nursing, using the self-care deficit nursing theory as a guide.

TABLE 10.1 Budget Elements

Costs	Processes	Revenues
Patient requirements for service	Basic staffing for service	General services (room revenue)
Staff requirements	Advanced or clinical services (over routine care)	Special services
To deliver service	Management: supervision, recruitment, planning, and programming	Percentage of goods sold, rentals
As employees		
For development	Education:	
Support services (unit management, secretarial)	Internal—orientation and inservice	
Equipment and supplies:	External	
Repair and maintenance	Affiliations, meetings, workshops (continuing education)	
Preventive maintenance		
Capital equipment	Advancement—formal education assistance	
Facilities—office space and indirect costs	Research and development	
	Goods—rental or sold	

Summary

In this chapter, the contribution of nursing theory to fiscal management and the delivery of safe, effective nursing is discussed. As described in previous chapters, nursing theory helps to define the domain and boundaries of nursing. This is an essential component in costing out nursing. Costs of many activities and procedures attributed to nursing are not initiated by nurses or carried out for nursing purposes. For example, O'Brien-Pallas et al. (1997) showed that rescheduling work to accommodate unanticipated events and delays caused by others has a major impact on nursing. These components of nursing work are "invisible" and do not appear in the costing system.

Accounting departments establish coding systems and allocate these codes to components of service delivery to determine costs. The components of service delivery are people, systems, equipment, and space. Although the coding systems may be common, there is little standardization in the implementation of definitions across accounting departments. Specifically, there is little standardization in determining which costs should be allocated to nursing.

Self-care deficit nursing theory can have a major impact on the utilization of resources. It provides direction for specifying nursing outcomes and developing a clinical information system that can include a database related to those outcomes. These data can then be linked to resource use and the budgeting process.

References

Androwich, I., & Stoupa, R. (1994). Count what counts: Information needs for nursing managers. *Seminars for Nurse Managers, 1*(2), 85-91.

Canavan, K. (1997). ANA study links nurse staffing to quality. Washington, D.C. *American Nurse, 29*(3), 1, 3.

Cockerill, R., & O'Brien-Pallas, L. L. (1990). Satisfaction with nursing workload systems. Report of a survey of Canadian hospitals, part A. *Canadian Journal of Nursing Administration, 3*(2), 17-22.

Cockerill, R., O'Brien-Pallas, L. L., Bolley, H., & Pink, G. (1993). Measuring nursing workload for case costing. *Nursing Economics$, 11*, 342-349.

Donlevey, H., & Pietruch, B. (1996). The connection delivery model: Reengineering nursing to provide care across the continuum. *Nursing Administration Quarterly, 20*(3), 73-78.

Edwardson, S. R., & Giovanetti, P. B. (1987). A review of cost-accounting methods for nursing services. *Nursing Economics$, 5*(3), 107-117.

Flarey, D. L. (1990). A methodology for costing nursing services. *Nursing Administration Quarterly, 14*(13), 41-51.

Gardner, K., Allhusen, J., Kamm, J., & Tobin, J. (1997). Determining the cost of care through clinical pathways. *Nursing Economics$, 15*, 213-217.

Halloran, E. (1985). Nursing workload, medical diagnosis related group and nursing diagnosis. *Research in Nursing and Health, 8*, 421-423.

Jelinek, R. (1967, Fall-Winter). A structured model for the patient care operation. *Health Services Research*, pp. 226-242.

Milholland, K. (1992). Naming what we do: Nursing vocabularies and databases. *Journal of American Health Information Management Association, 63*(10), 58-61.

O'Brien-Pallas, L. L., Irvine, D., Peereboom, E., & Murray, M. (1997). Measuring nursing workload: Understanding the variability. *Nursing Economics$, 15*, 171-182.

Pinkerton, S. E. (1996). Development of a new nursing organization model. *Nursing Economics$, 14*, 197-204.

Sherman, J. J. (1990). Costs of nursing care: A review. *Nursing Admininistration Quarterly, 14*(3), 11-17.

Utilization of Nursing Personnel

Maximizing utilization of nursing personnel involves matching the nursing needs of the target population with nursing resources in such a way that cost-effective service is provided for the population and for individuals within that population. This is a challenge. Without a shared mental model to provide direction for defining the domain and boundaries of nursing and articulation of nursing with other health care professionals in the enterprise, it is an impossibility. It can be a source of frustration and misunderstanding among nurses and between nurses and non-nurse administrators. In this chapter, the interrelationship of population descriptions, nursing capabilities, and utilization of nursing personnel is discussed.

Many studies have been done to try to determine the benefits and costs of different methods for delivery of nursing that involve both licensed and non-licensed nursing personnel, such as primary nursing and team nursing. A study by Mark (1992) suggested that there is no "best" model for delivery of nursing and that the focus should therefore be on "the core of care"—the patient (p. 62). Yet in redesign, the focus has tended to be on nursing roles and types of workers rather than on developing a way of thinking about nursing, operationalizing a nursing theory in practice, facilitating its use, and defining and evaluating nursing outcomes. This is work that needs to be done. Self-care deficit nursing theory can be a useful tool toward these ends.

TABLE 11.1 Nursing Considerations in Use of Health Care Resources

Self-Care Systems in Operation	Questions on Transitions: Admission, Transfer, Discharge	Decisions About Use of Health Care Resources
Self-care	Health status/self-care	Ambulatory care—MD offices,
Self/dependent	status—maintain/protect,	clinics, HMOs, nurse centers,
care	improve, regress	surgicenters, etc.
Self/dependent/	Type/amount of help/services	Personal care home
nursing care	needed	Retirement community—full
	Location of delivery—	service
	eligibility, length of	Day care
	stay/service	Home health
	Available personal	Nursing home
	resources—social, financial	Hospice
	Environment—physical, social,	Acute care hospital—emergency
	cultural, urban, suburban, rural	department, inpatient service
	Community support systems—	(community, tertiary specialty)
	transportation, meals on wheels,	
	churches, etc.	
	Costs	

Considerations in Use of Health Care Resources

In Table 11.1, the factors to be considered in the use of health care resources are identified. The basis for decision making is the self-care system(s) in operation in reference to the recipient(s) of the service. Areas of questioning associated with decisions about admission, discharge, and transfer of persons from one resource to another are suggested along with the health care service to be accessed.

In each of the health care resources listed in Table 11.1, the nature and extent of actual or potential dependency in self-care need to be anticipated. (Note that nursing is the predominant service in almost all of the health care resources, with the possible exceptions of personal care homes and day care, where nursing may or may not be involved.)

When daily self/dependent care is considered in relationship to the types of health care resources available, the questions that need to be answered about admittance, transfer, and discharge from one resource to another must take into consideration what persons can or cannot do and what type of assistance is needed, particularly nursing. For example, some people go into comprehensive retirement communities seeking protection and security in the event they will not be able to manage some aspects of their lives in general and their health care in particular when they get older. Nursing is an integral component in that these institutions offer assisted care and nursing home care. Other people may prefer to let things happen and make alternative decisions when the need arises. Managed-care providers are becoming more involved in these decisions. They are concerned not only about the use of health care resources, such as reducing expensive emergency room visits and readmissions to hospitals, but also about how safely and effectively individuals can manage on their own or with appropriate assistance.

Nursing systems need to be designed to address the anticipated self-care abilities and limitations of groups and populations of patients for each level of care or health care resource. The concept of centralization of planning for admissions, discharge, and transfers from one institution to another may rest with the managed-care provider (payer) rather than a particular institution. On the other hand, a hospital or other health care agency, particularly one that offers a range of health care services on the continuum of care, might examine what the typical trajectory of care would be for particular patient population groups. Cost estimates can be made for both patients and the health care agency in relation to choice of options and cost control under a capitation arrangement. Patient dependency in self-care and dependent care become key variables in planning. A knowledgeable and experienced advanced nursing practitioner should be involved, taking a leading role in this activity and helping to determine how best to utilize nursing resources to meet general health goals and the purposes of the health care enterprise. Self-care deficit nursing theory can provide direction to the advanced nursing practitioner.

Nursing Agency

In self-care deficit nursing theory, Orem (1995) clearly delineated the role of the nurse as she introduced the construct of nursing agency. This she defined as

> the developed capabilities of persons educated as nurses that empower them to represent themselves as nurse and within the frame of a legitimate interpersonal relationship to act, to know, and to help persons in such relationships to meet their therapeutic self-care demands and to regulate the development or exercise of their self-care agency. (p. 458)

She went on to say that mature persons with this specialized knowledge "master the cognitive and practical operations of nursing practice" under the guidance of advanced nursing practitioners and, through varied clinical nursing experiences, learn to provide nursing to persons representing some range of types of nursing cases (p. 247). Nursing agency varies as a consequence of basic conditioning factors affecting the nurse: education, experience, personal attributes, interests, and sociocultural factors. Opportunities for varied work experiences, availability of employment in different health care situations, and organizational commitment (or lack thereof) to promote and facilitate the nurse's growth and development in practice are all factors contributing to the development of nursing agency.

A variety of legislation controls the practice of nursing, the use of the term *registered nurse,* and the education of persons who call themselves nurses. But despite such legislation, there is still confusion in society about registered nurses, licensed practical nurses, nursing assistants, nursing aides, and physician assistants, all of whom may be performing tasks that appear to be similar. Education for this work related to "nursing" may vary from on-the-job training to preparation at the doctoral level.

In many situations, the question arises as to whether the person called "nurse" is fully functioning as a nurse or fulfilling some other role using the nurse's diversified knowledge and skills. For example, as a nurse case manager, the nurse may be acting as an agent of a health care provider or insurance company whose primary function is to coordinate health care services for cost efficiency and cost-effectiveness purposes. Little actual nursing of patients and families may take place. Another example is the nurse practitioner who primarily functions as a physician extender and focuses on the medical aspects of care. The nursing component may be limited and not developed to an advanced level. In both situations, adequate or optimal provision of nursing cannot be ensured. The nurse may not be fully functioning as a nurse. Similarly, the nurse administrator may focus primarily on the management component and have little to do with nursing per se or with leading in the development of nursing practice.

From the opposite perspective, a recurring issue for the nursing profession is the use of nurse extenders: not extenders of medicine, as described above, but persons with little or no education in nursing and with limited knowledge and skills to provide nursing care. Nursing assistants with on-the-job and/or some vocational training in nursing have long served as nurse extenders under nursing supervision in various health care situations. The current concern is the hiring of nonlicensed personnel by health care institutions to provide nursing (and other services) and replace licensed nurses in order to reduce costs. As a result, at a time when registered nurses are having to care for more acutely ill patients, their time, energies, and skills for providing nursing to patients may be diluted and diverted by having to supervise increased numbers of less skilled workers.

Differentiated Nursing Practice

The organization and use of nursing personnel to achieve nursing results and delineate nursing's contribution to the health care team requires creative planning and cooperative endeavor among a variety of nursing personnel and with nursing administration. Nursing practice can be differentiated by education, experience, and competence. Education and experience are fairly straightforward criteria to identify and measure. Competence is more complicated.

Competence must not only address technical skill in performance of procedures but relate to the process components of diagnosis, prescription, design, planning, and production. The content of these process components is derived from the mental model in use. Levels of competence in relation to the process steps can be specified when the content associated with each step is known, as illustrated in the following discussion.

All nursing personnel need to know and understand the basic tenets and concepts of the mental model or theory in use. However, administration must recognize that all categories of personnel providing services related to nursing are not able to exercise the same degree of judgment and skill. For example, when self-care deficit nursing theory is providing direction for nursing practice, a nursing assistant may understand that patients are to be encouraged to function as independently as possible in self-care. Consequently, early in the morning an elderly stroke patient is encouraged to do as much as possible. By the end of the day, however, fatigue and decreased endurance may limit the person's action capabilities and add to his or her enervation. Nursing assistants who fail to recognize this may continue to routinely urge the patient to make an effort when it is inappropriate and possibly unsafe. In such instances, the registered nurse responsible for the patient should assess the situation and intervene to supplement or complement for the patient's lack of ability at that time. Danger lies in routinizing care to such a degree that individual patient differences in abilities and preferences are not recognized and dealt with. Reduction in employment of registered nurses and use of nonlicensed personnel to reduce costs places patients potentially at risk. About a 60:40 ratio of licensed to unlicensed staff is reasonable in a less acute health care service such as rehabilitation. (This is in contrast to the staff mix for acute medical surgical units of 70% RNs to 30% nursing assistants, as reported by Sovie, 1995.) Otherwise, the increased supervisory span for the registered nurses dilutes their time for direct care. In these situations also, the informal organization may take over from the formal. Patient care suffers, nurse turnover increases, and little is saved.

All nurses today are taught the nursing process, interpersonal techniques, and methods of communication with and about patients. The depth of understanding of the self-care deficit nursing theory and the creative insights and experience of the nurse will dictate how well the nurse identifies nursing problems in terms of self-care deficits, limitations in self-care abilities (and dependent care abilities if appropriate), the factors causing or influencing them, and how to manage them. The largest proportion of registered nurses today are associate-degree graduates. Though technically competent with some scientific knowledge to understand and use validated reliable nursing technologies, these nurses need professionally prepared advanced practitioners to guide and support them and to develop and validate nursing technologies and nursing systems for individual patients and groups of patients with whom they work.

Advanced Practitioners of Nursing

In the past, definitions of the advanced nursing practitioner's role emphasized teaching and counseling but not about what, except to say that the nurse should take a "holistic" and "caring" approach. The "what" may be seen primarily as the patient's need to follow the medically prescribed regimen and to maintain or attain health. But this does not look at all the other factors as they influence persons' abilities to meet their care demands. A nursing examination should address the self-care requisites to be met, the foundational capabilities, the power components, and the self-care operations needed to meet the action demands and require nurses to identify what and how various basic conditioning factors affect each of these and the person's system of daily living (see Chapter 2 and Chapter 4's Appendix 4A). This assessment requires as extensive a workup as a medical examination, if not more extensive in some aspects. In-depth knowledge of the medical component being dealt with better enables the advanced practitioner to anticipate and plan ways with patients to meet their therapeutic self-care demands and to recognize how a medical condition and/or its therapy may affect all of this.

Nurse practitioners, with their medical knowledge and skills, are in increasing demand in both primary and acute care to relieve overburdened physicians. Advanced practitioners of nursing with this knowledge and skill, functioning in direct practice, manage and coordinate the care of individual patients as their units of service. The value of these practitioners will increase as their nursing role is strengthened to more clearly and definitively deal with why patients and families are or are not able to adhere to a therapeutic regimen. The scope of practice of the advanced practitioner is broadened not only by knowing the nursing variables of therapeutic self-care demand and self-care agency but by having the structure to identify what and how basic conditioning factors other than and along with the medical ones affect these persons and their management of self/dependent care. Some advanced practitioners of nursing may follow their patients not only on an outpatient basis but in the hospital, nursing homes, and patients' homes if needed. The size of the caseload of the advanced practitioners will depend on the range of care provided.

Advanced practitioners of nursing habitually think and function from a nursing theoretical perspective. They use nursing theory in conjunction with comprehensive antecedent knowledge and extensive clinical experience, incorporating new nursing knowledge and knowledge from related fields to develop and improve nursing practice for the benefit of patients/clients, nursing, and health services. The addition of medical knowledge and skills provides a firm foundation for understanding the demands, effects, and results of the health condition and its therapy on self/dependent care (Geden & Taylor, 1996). Knowledge generated by psychologists is frequently used by the advanced practitioner. For example, Backscheider (1974) looked at self-care requirements and self-care capacities of an inner-city, largely black, diabetic patient population to determine their level of operative knowing as conceptualized by Piaget. This aided selection and/or development of more appropriate, effective, and efficient teaching and assisting methodologies.

The Nurse Case Manager

The case manager role for the advanced practitioner of nursing focuses on the overall care management of a caseload of patients provided by nurses and other health care providers. This may be limited to a hospital episode of care that cuts across geographic areas or services in the hospital or may extend beyond hospital walls to address the whole continuum of care in the community. The case manager collaborates with other health team members in seeking to coordinate the care provided and the resources used. There may be a case manager in each setting and perhaps one overall who coordinates the care between settings. The model at Carondelet St. Mary's Hospital and Health Center in Tucson, Arizona, addresses continuity of care by offering a range of services. Nursing case management extends to long-term care, home health, hospice, clinics, and nursing centers. Nursing is reported to be a major contributor to the profit margin of the hospital. This program, moreover, is one of the few in the country to be identified as nursing theory based. Margaret Newman's theory of health as expanding consciousness is used (Cohen, & Cesta, 1997; Lamb, 1992; Michaels, 1991; Newman, Lamb, & Michaels, 1991). Many descriptions of nursing outcomes in these articles relate to self-care. It is not clear from these articles, however, how Newman's theory is used to structure nursing practice or delineate the use of nursing personnel.

Advanced nurses who function at the scientific level of practice should maintain the nursing focus—how self/dependent care systems are being managed—no matter what their role or function may be. This includes providing direct care or serving as case managers to maintain cost control and to ensure quality of care in collaboration and coordination with health care team members within an institution or across the continuum of care. As researchers and developers, they may be responsible for the design, development, and evaluation of nursing systems and new nursing technologies and approaches. In all of these roles, a clear concept of nursing's role and contribution to health care is essential.

Differentiation Between Basic and Advanced Levels of Nurse Functioning

When using a theoretical framework such as self-care deficit nursing theory, one can make a distinction between the level of functioning of a basic nurse and that of an advanced practitioner of nursing. Table 11.2 shows the differences in level of functioning. It is apparent that the basic nurse needs the leadership and guidance of the advanced nurse in developing both nursing knowledge and nursing practice.

An Example of Using an Advanced Practitioner to Facilitate Program Development

Appendix 11A presents extracts from minutes of two meetings between an advanced practitioner of nursing operating from a nursing theory base and two staff nurses, experienced baccalaureate graduates functioning as specialists in enterostomy/wound care. These minutes demonstrate how an advanced nursing practitioner working from the perspective of nursing theory can help staff nurses who may or may not be familiar with theory to analyze the characteristics of the group of patients they deal with, explore nursing resources available, identify patient outcomes, specify problem areas, and design a care system to improve services to the population of concern. It is evident from the data given that these nurses are intelligent, knowledgeable about their patients, perceptive, caring, and creative in seeking and finding ways to assist the patients and their families with minimal organizational support. They deal not only with the physical care but with the personal and interpersonal aspects trying out a variety of ways to assist patients and caregivers to manage as effectively as possible even under severely limiting conditions. These nurses function independently in a large teaching health care institution that encompasses hospital inpatient, outpatient, and nursing home care. Home health is used by referral. Their problem is how best to structure their work to improve care and be more effective in the processes of care. The advanced nursing practitioner with management knowledge and skill as well as in-depth knowledge of the self-care deficit nursing theory is helping them to do this by beginning with where they are and working through them to build for the future.

Although these two nurses have no formal knowledge of the self-care deficit nursing theory, what they described about their patients can be easily organized within the framework of the theory. The theory then serves as a basis for examining, analyzing, and developing a practice model with them. The model, when developed, should help to improve the care provided and the system of service while reducing costs to the hospital. Clearly, much needs to be done, including procuring support from nursing administration to achieve some of these nurses' goals, such as developing a nurse clinic and obtaining clerical support and supplies. The advanced practitioner in the role of consultant seeks to help them perceive the range of work that needs to be done and organize, analyze, plan, and develop their practice and a system of care. The advanced practitioner can also help them develop nursing diagnostic technologies and documentation methods or forms to ensure consistency and completeness in recording their care and its results so that they work within the present system more effectively. At present, with no framework to organize their practice and to clarify their concerns, these nurses experience a high level of frustration.

In a not dissimilar instance some years ago, one of us helped to develop a nurse-conducted clinic for diabetic patients and for other types of patients as

TABLE 11.2 Differentiating the Basic Nurse From the Advanced Practice Nurse

Basic Nurse	Advanced Practice Nurse
Has fundamental knowledge of nursing practice and related theory	Has broader, more in-depth knowledge of nursing practice and related theory
Practice relies heavily on rules, procedures; tends to focus on selected aspects of situation; limited conceptualization of the whole.	Practices from a conceptualization of the whole, focusing on the immediate situation within the broader context of the whole.
May or may not be aware of mental model directing practice. Models that have been learned have not been internalized, and nurses are dependent on continuing support for model in the work environment.	Consistently operates from a specific theoretical framework including social, interpersonal, and technological dimensions.
Uses standardized nursing technologies to identify/label common overt nursing problems in the nursing process and implement nursing prescriptions.	Describes patient populations from a theoretical perspective, testing and validating in area of specialty practice with patient populations. Provides direct care and nursing consultation.
Focus is on practice for individual patients:	Focus is on continuing development and improvement of nursing practice for patient populations:
Seeks nursing consultation for care of complex patients.	Designs and develops nursing systems for patient populations, consults with nursing administration.

well (Allison, 1973). The nurse practicing in the diabetic clinic commented, "You never told me what to do. You helped me to do what I knew I should be doing for patients and do it better, but I didn't know how to go about it." This is a role that an advanced practitioner can play in relation to staff nurses. It is a team relationship. The staff nurse gives feedback on whether something is working, and together the staff nurse and advanced practitioner plan and try new or different approaches. A nurse administrator in this role with a well-developed conceptualization of nursing can provide leadership, guidance, and support to practicing nurses, helping them to work within the health care system to give better care to more patients in a cost-effective way. This also helps to develop strong nurses. They come to know and understand more fully their domain of practice; thus, nurse satisfaction and nurse retention increase. Where nurses have a sense of growth and self-worth, they are more productive for themselves and the organization.

TABLE 11.2 *Continued*

Basic Nurse	*Advanced Practice Nurse*
Participates in nursing studies.	Collaborates with nursing administration in planning for delivery of nursing.
Continues scholarly work, utilizes literature, analyzes own practice.	Develops, tests, and evaluates nursing diagnostic and treatment technologies, nursing documentation, and new/improved approaches for provision of care to individuals and patients.
Evaluates outcomes of own work with individual patients.	Evaluates outcomes of practice for groups of patients.
Coordinates and collaborates with other health care team members in provision of care to individual patients.	Conducts nursing studies and identifies and formalizes nursing knowledge—exploring, developing, and refining concepts in the theory.
May teach others (patients/families/nursing personnel) depending on his or her understanding of the theory.	Continues own study; publishes.
	Coordinates and collaborates with other health care disciplines in design of systems of care, planning, and provision of care to groups of patients.
	Formally serves as a role model for other nurses in the use of the theory

Population Descriptions: A Tool in Determining Utilization of Nursing Personnel

In Chapter 4, processes and descriptive categories relative to defining patient populations were introduced. As discussed in Chapters 4 and 6, defining/ describing patient populations is a precursor to designing health-related programs and associated nursing services for those populations. In acute care hospital settings, nursing is frequently thought of in relation to the medical service being offered, such as psychiatry, obstetrics, and surgery. In community settings, the service is frequently organized around age groups, settings such as home care or place of employment, or health states such as sexually transmitted disease. Self-care deficit nursing theory provides a more precise way of considering the need for nursing—in relation to the nature of the self-care deficit—with the medical service, age group, setting, and health state all acting as conditioning factors. When the population is viewed from this perspective—that is, the characteristics of the self-care deficit—the nursing required becomes a function of the nature of the existing or potential self-care deficit (the "core of care" referred to by Mark, 1992) and falls into three major categories: wholly compensatory, in which patients/clients are unable to carry out any of their self-care; partly compensatory; and supportive-educative.

Developing and delivering a nursing program for a population includes determining the need, designing the service, providing the service, and evaluating it. The educational preparation, knowledge, and skills for each of these steps vary from those of an advanced practitioner educated at the graduate level to those of a nursing aide working under the supervision of a registered nurse. The rationale for the educational preparation required and category of worker assigned to provide the services should be a function of patient need, not of the particular tasks being performed. For example, although technically proficient, many nurses prepared in associate-degree programs do not have the knowledge, skill, and experience to assess patients to determine their needs for nursing and to design systems of nursing care. To this end, we are proposing that within any nursing service, consideration should be given to differentiating nursing practice relative to patient need for nursing and educational preparation and capabilities of the nurse as well as the characteristics of the target population.

Nursing Systems and Patient Populations

■ *Wholly Compensatory Nursing Systems*

Persons incapacitated by medical or surgical conditions requiring wholly compensatory nursing systems may or may not be able to participate in the decision making about the care required. When patients are unable to participate, in addition to the skills associated with monitoring and regulating sophisticated technologies, nurses must establish systems of communication with the patients and with the families. In the midst of managing the machines and attending to physical needs, the nurses must maintain the nursing focus, including promotion of development; overcoming of factors interfering with development; and anticipating, projecting, and compensating for what persons can, cannot, and/or should not do. Without a theory of nursing practice such as self-care deficit nursing theory to provide direction for nursing practice and construction of standards and care maps, nurses tend to revert to practicing from the dominant model in place, the medical model, resulting in performance of procedures and carrying out of policies without a framework for attending to the whole person. Care maps that are developed in these settings tend to reflect the concerns of medicine with little direction to nurses for carrying out the less visible tasks of nursing. Advanced nursing practitioners are needed in these situations to design wholly compensatory nursing systems, to supervise the practitioners implementing the planned systems, and to evaluate the effectiveness of the systems. Their knowledge and skills may also be required for developing capabilities of family members and nursing personnel in carrying out the required care.

The advanced nursing practitioner working from the perspective of self-care deficit nursing theory will attend not just to the treatment/procedure/task but to all of the variables identified in Figure 2.4 as significant to the execution of self-care. This type of proactive nursing service can result in lower costs to the overall system because complications can be prevented.

For example, an advanced practitioner who began working from a self-care deficit nursing theory perspective that provided a framework for looking at developmental issues noted that in the population of young people who became quadriplegic following an accident, development appeared to be arrested at the age at which the accident occurred. This arrested development resulted in behavioral problems such as inappropriate attention seeking; acting out in the form of risk-taking behavior, including substance abuse; and being just plain difficult to work with and abusive to personnel. When strategies were put in place to deal with the developmental delay, the amount of nursing time required in working with this group of patients was decreased. In addition, when it was recognized that the issues related to development were fairly widespread but had a similar origin, it was possible to deal with them on a group level. This is considerably less costly than providing this service on a one-to-one basis.

■ *Partly Compensatory Nursing Systems*

An example of designing of a partly compensatory nursing system for a population of spinal cord injury patients in which various levels of nursing personnel are utilized is presented in Chapter 6, Appendix 6A. The role of the clinical nurse specialist included identifying the particular characteristics from which the population description was developed, participating in developing the standards of care that provided direction for day-to-day management of this population, evaluating the effectiveness of the program, and acting as a resource to staff for managing individual and populationwide problems. In this design for spinal cord injury patients, the RN was responsible for a designated number of patients from time of admission through discharge: doing a complete workup on admission; designing, planning, and providing care as needed from the RN and others; and following up throughout the patient's hospitalization to discharge. RNs also served as team leaders, assigning nursing personnel—new RNs, licensed practical nurses, and nursing assistants—according to their knowledge and skill level to perform various activities of care and supervising them as necessary. These nursing personnel performed routine aspects of care, made and documented observations of patients, and reported pertinent observations to the RN responsible for the patients. The charge nurse (RN) oversaw the functioning of the various teams, assigning personnel, providing assistance as needed and managing the coordination and communications systems for effective operation in the health care system, including staffing schedules of nursing personnel.

■ Supportive-Educative Nursing Systems

Supportive-educative nursing systems have long been the mode of operation in traditional community health nursing, where the emphasis has been on prevention—prenatal teaching programs, parenting programs, and the like. In the 1950s, progressive patient care was advocated, and a number of hospitals had self-care units. These ceased to exist when the demand for acute care beds increased. Today, as unused acute care beds have become available in some institutions, short-stay units have been opened in which patients and families assume much responsibility for their own care. Nurse staffing may be limited to one registered nurse as primary nurse and a few nursing assistants. Patient education is emphasized through use of written materials and teaching. ("Cooperative Care," 1985; Wallace, 1986). Two such models, one in a veterans' hospital and another in a tertiary teaching hospital, base the care on Orem's self-care deficit nursing theory (Lott, Blazey, & West, 1992; Weis, 1985). The supportive-educative nursing system generally pertains in these situations.

In another example of a supportive-educative nursing system in the current health care environment, RNs are assuming considerable responsibility for telephone triage and are able to handle a variety of patient problems. The nurses have depth of knowledge about the clinical specialty area. For example, on a cardiac service, an RN using medical protocols analyzes the information provided by the caller and makes decisions about what to advise persons with regard to the identified (or unidentified) medical problem. Critical to the nurse's decisions should be knowledge about what the patient or caregiver is doing (or not doing) to manage the self-care system in relation to the patient's condition and the prescribed medical regimen. Good nurses may automatically do this. In general, this will not happen without a systematic consistent way of inquiring about and analyzing information in reference to the total management of self-care. If the patient fails to manage his or her condition and treatment, the medical regimen is not handled properly. The patient may get into trouble. The problem may be due not to the prescribed medical treatment or condition but to how the patient/caregiver is handling the situation.

The early work of Backscheider (1974) illustrates that being effective in promoting self-care through a supportive-educative system is much more complex than providing educational materials, teaching, or giving advice. On the basis of observations made with a diabetic population, the author listed the multitude of capabilities required to identify self-care requirements and to perform self-care. Current health promotion literature supports the observations of Backscheider.

Model for Delivery of Nursing Across the Continuum of Care

At present, the self-care perspective needs to be extended from care in one location to care across a continuum, with transitions from one health care environment to another. Definitive input will be needed by nursing administration and other nursing personnel for the design, development, and implementation of nursing systems for the continuum of care. Close estimation of costs of nursing personnel needed to ensure quality of care at each stage and level is essential to effective management of resources.

In the traditional trajectory of health care, a patient simply goes from home to a doctor or clinic and in acute situations goes to an emergency room and then may be admitted to a hospital. On discharge from the hospital, the person returns home, with follow-up in a doctor's office or clinic. Variations in this process include use of a home health service or a referral to a nursing home for a short or an indefinite period of time. Other community resources may be needed. Individuals have the right to choose, some of which may depend on their economic means. With managed care through case management, the focus is on helping persons to use the most economical resources along the whole trajectory of care. The case manager enters into the decision making with the patient, family, and physician.

Nursing criteria are needed to help define and spell out in various care maps for inpatient, outpatient, and home health services factors to identify the need, eligibility, process, and outcomes of care. These should relate to entry, continuing care, and discharge from a service. These decisions are not made solely on the medical condition and its treatment. The interrelationship of all of the variables of concern to nursing as identified in Figure 2.4 need to be considered, along with the types and capabilities of nurses' knowledge and skills needed to meet these requirements in different settings and the best setting to meet the needs. Some approximation should be made of costs in terms of outcomes desired or possible. Advanced practitioners of nursing can help identify and formalize the potential nursing required in each health care setting and the relationships of one to the other and to other health care resources. A model depicting delivery of nursing across the continuum is shown in Table 11.3.

The communication system is critical to any plans to coordinate nursing and other health care services across the continuum of care. Delineation of the information required for each stage of care is needed. Attention should be given to inputs requiring rapid response, reduction of redundance in data collected, and prevention of information overload. In the model, criteria for determining nursing needs for a patient population are suggested. These variables identified in the criteria are a reiteration of the variables identified in Chapter 4's Appendix 4A. A potential direction of patient flow to and from various health care resources is set forth from three perspectives—the patients' place of residence, ambulatory care services, and institutional care. Note that comprehensive retirement communities generally offer a range of health care services except for hospital care and perhaps visits to specialty physicians. Nursing systems for different patient populations in different settings and transitions between them need to be designed and developed. When this work has been completed, a nurse case manager using these criteria may oversee a large group of patients in each setting and/or across settings.

Raiwet, Halliwell, Andruski, and Wilson (1997) reported on the leadership of nursing in designing a care map that provided for a seamless continuum of care between hospital and community. In this case, the standards were not limited to a particular health care agency but addressed the entire episode of care from initial contact with a health care service through inpatient care, ending at time of discharge from community-based home care. Undoubtedly, this type of care mapping across the trajectory of the illness episode, including services by several agencies, will be the mapping of the future. Such care maps require that the self-care requirements of patients and the requirements for nursing be clearly delineated, for these are essential components of the decision making for transfer, design of care required, and evaluation of effectiveness of services provided.

TABLE 11.3 Model for Delivery of Nursing Across the Continuum of Care

Nursing Criteria for Decision Making	Patients' Living Environment (Supportive-Educative Care)	Ambulatory Services (Supportive-Educative or Partly Compensatory Care)	Institutional Health (Supportive-Educative, Partly Compensatory, or Wholly Compensatory Care)
Calculate TSCD	Home—self/ dependent care	MD office, clinic, surgicenter, nurse clinic, etc. (N)	Hospital: emergency, general, specialty (psychiatric, rehabilitation, etc.) (N)
Estimate self/ dependent care	Home—personal care Retirement community (N)	Home health (N) Day care	
Estimate the values of the BCFs that are operational	Nursing home (N) Hospice (N)		
Stability/instability, acuity/chronicity of health state			
Complexity of Dx and Rx technologies			
Other			
Estimate the extent/ urgency of other health services needed			
Assess environment— physical, social, cultural			
Specify type/amount of nursing needed Estimate costs			

▲————————————————▲————————————————▲
Nursing Care Management Across the Continuum of Care

NOTE: (N) denotes service areas where nursing is provided. BCF, basic conditioning factor; TSCD, therapeutic self-care demand.

An example of a set of criteria for transitions from one health care setting to another based on requirements for nursing is given in Table 11.4. This table demonstrates how a publicly funded home health care agency used the structure provided by the theory to determine admission/discharge criteria for nursing services. An extract of the patient classification system and criteria for admission

TABLE 11.4 Home Care Nursing Priorities

Type I: Wholly Compensatory: Nurse or significant other is acting for the patient. Medium priority for admission.

Subtype I: Patient is unable to control position and movement, unresponsive to stimuli, unable to monitor environment and to convey information.

Methods of Helping: Do for, protect

Admission/Discharge: Assess and discharge to appropriate facility or to palliative care program. Accepted to home care only if wait listed for facility care or end stage palliative care.

Subtype II: Patient is aware and can make observations, judgements, and decisions about self-care but cannot or should not perform actions.

Methods of Helping: Do for, regulate environment, provide environment that supports development, teach

Admission/Discharge: Patients should not be discharged until other resources are in place to provide ongoing emotional support and/or protection.

Subtype III: Patient is unable to attend to self or make judgements or decisions but is ambulatory and able to do some self-care with guidance, support, and supervision.

Methods of Helping: Do for, guide and direct, provide physical and psychological support, maintain an environment that supports development.

Admission/Discharge: Medium priority for admission. Accepted to home care only if wait-listed for alternate care or assessment.

Type II: Partially Compensatory: Patient has a medical problem and lacks knowledge or skill to perform related activities. May not be physically able or psychologically ready to do tasks or learn at present. High priority for admission.

Methods of Helping: Combination of do for, guide, support, teach, provide developmental environment.

Admission/Discharge: Reassess every 2 weeks.

Type III: Educational-Supportive: Patient is able to perform or can and should learn to perform required care. Requirements are for help in decision making, behavior change or control, acquisition of knowledge or skills.

Methods of Helping: Guide, support, teach, provide developmental environment.

SOURCE: Material reprinted courtesy of the Vancouver/Richmond Health Board, Vancouver, Canada.

and discharge are provided. Persons falling outside of these criteria but still wanting to be cared for at home would be referred to a private home care nursing service.

Job Descriptions and Performance Appraisal

A question that legitimately might be asked is whether the use of nursing theory should be incorporated into the job description and evaluated on the performance appraisal of the practicing nurse. If a theory of nursing has been accepted as the substantive basis for practice to ensure consistency in focus and a common basis for thinking and communicating about nursing in the institution, then the answer logically is "yes." In Chapter 9 in the discussion of standards of nursing practice, the performance appraisal system was identified as the place where achievement of the expected standards in relation to practice would be evaluated. When nurses are recruited and employed by an enterprise, the nursing theory being used and expected of them should be explained so that the nurse understands this expectation from the outset before making a final decision about accepting employment. By the same token, the agency or institution has an obligation to provide an educational program and opportunities for clinical experience for development in practice that is consistent with the identified standards.

Job descriptions for each level of nursing worker should incorporate expectations about how the mental model or nursing theory should be reflected in practice. Items might include critical thinking in nursing diagnoses and management of nursing cases, teaching of patients/families about self/dependent care, teaching of other nurses about the theory, and case analyses in patient conferences. Promotion to a higher level position may be conditioned on evidence of advanced understanding of self-care and nursing theory and evidence of use of this understanding in provision of patient services or in support of other nursing staff. Where theory-based practice is operational, nurses tend to seek further education because they recognize more clearly what they know and do not know about nursing of patients. Further educational preparation, in turn, enhances their performance and potential for job promotion.

The overall performance of nursing staff in practice based on a theory of nursing such as the self-care deficit nursing theory should promote coherence and consistency in the nursing approach throughout a nursing department or agency. Nurses gain a clearer sense of identity and understanding about what nursing has to offer and how nursing relates to services and goals of others in the health care system. The productivity of nursing in terms of patient outcomes can be measured through process and outcome evaluation studies. In turn, the findings may be examined in relation to utilization of nursing resources: types and levels of personnel and costs, time, and level of performance of each nursing employee and of the department or health care program as a whole.

Evaluation of nursing practice is based on nursing documentation, oral and written reports, and observations of the nurse's performance. In discussion of nursing cases and in written documentation, does the nurse, for example, describe how the self-care system is affected by current health state and how self-care capabilities and limitations may affect the physician's plan of care or the work of other health care disciplines, teaching of patients and families, or teaching of other nurses? Discussion of the literature applicable to the patient situation and testing of hypotheses in a systematic, practical manner may be a way to evaluate the more advanced practitioner of nursing.

How the nurse is evaluated will depend on the system or form used by the institution, agency, or program. Some forms may be standardized in general structure to be applicable to all personnel. Criteria for the specific item areas in types of nursing behaviors desired, however, can be established by the particular institution. The mental model or theory of nursing can provide direction for specifying these behaviors. If nursing standards of practice and of care are based on the self-care deficit nursing theory, they will provide another basis for establishing criteria for the performance appraisal.

Summary

Utilization of nursing personnel from a nursing theory perspective has been explored in this chapter. Use of self-care deficit nursing theory gives the administrator a broader perspective from which to make decisions about utilization of nursing personnel. The administrator reviews levels of functioning of nursing personnel to ensure that the social, interpersonal, and technological dimensions of patient requirements are met and that nursing results are achieved cost-effectively. The nurse's first focus, seeking to ascertain what persons have to know and do to manage their health care and their relevant abilities and inabilities, requires understanding of the multiple factors impinging on the situation. This is the role of the advanced practitioner of nursing. Task-oriented nursing personnel can be used effectively under the direction of theory-based practitioners of nursing who keep the nursing focus paramount. Expectations of nursing personnel from a nursing theory perspective can be spelled out through job descriptions and performance appraisal systems.

References

Allison, S. E. (1973). A framework for nursing action in a nurse conducted diabetic management clinic. *Journal of Nursing Administration, 3*(4), 53-60.

Backscheider, J. E. (1974). Self-care requirements, self-care capabilities, and nursing systems in the diabetic nurse management clinic. *American Journal of Public Health, 64,* 1138-1146.

Cohen, E. L., & Cesta, T. G. (1997). *Nursing case management: From concept to evaluation* (2nd ed.). St. Louis, MO: C. V. Mosby.

Cooperative care tied to quicker recovery. (1985). *Hospitals, 59*(23), 59-60.

Geden, E., & Taylor, S. G. (1996). How is nursing expressed by nurse practitioners in the primary health care setting. *International Orem Society Newsletter, 5*(2), 9-11.

Lamb, G. S. (1992). Conceptual and methodological issues in nurse case management records. *Advances in Nursing Science, 15*(2), 16-24.

Lott, T. F., Blazey, M. E., & West, M. G. (1992). Patient participation in health care: An underused resource. *Nursing Clinics of North America, 27*(1), 61-76.

Mark, B. A. (1992). Characteristics of nursing practice models. *Journal of Nursing Administration, 22*(11), 77-85.

Michaels, C. (1991). Carondelet St. Mary's nursing enterprise. *Nursing Clinics of North America, 27*(1), 77-85.

Newman, M. A., Lamb, G. S., & Michaels, C. (1991). Nurse case management: The coming together of theory and practice. *Nursing and Health Care, 12,* 404-408.

Orem, D. E. (1995). *Nursing: Concepts of practice* (5th ed.). St. Louis, MO: Mosby Year-Book.

Raiwet, C., Halliwell, G., Andruski, L., & Wilson, D. (1997, January). Care maps across the continuum. *Canadian Nurse,* pp. 26-30.

Sovie, M. D. (1995). Tailoring hospitals for managed care and integrated health systems. *Nursing Economics$, 13,* 72-83.

Wallace, C. (1986). Hospital's "personalized" care unit may boost share, patient satisfaction. *Modern Healthcare, 16*(1), 36, 38.

Weis, A. (1985). Cooperative care: An application of Orem's self-care theory. *Patient Education and Counseling, 11,* 141-146.

Extracts From Minutes Describing a Patient Population, a Nursing System for It, and Organizational Problems

Initial Meeting

Purpose

To design and develop a nursing system for wound, enterostomal, and incontinent patients.

Description of Patient Population Served

1. Basic conditioning factors—general characteristics
   1.1. Age: Newborns to elderly/terminal; predominantly older with chronic wounds.
   1.2. Developmental stage: Varied.
   1.3. Race: about 60% black, remainder white.
   1.4. Sex: Males and females; young black males—20% gunshot wounds; females—diverticulitis, cancer—pelvic exenteration.
   1.5. Education: 80% less than 12th grade, operational level of majority about 6th grade. This does not interfere with teaching: Use pictures, practice doing. Example: An illiterate mechanic understood gaskets, stoma appliance related to a

gasket. This was easily understood. Use patient's language, if necessary (e.g., "shit" instead of "stool"). Lay terminology the patients understand works best.

1.6. Socioeconomic status: Majority on Medicaid, Medicare, no pay, 20% potential insurance. No money for supplies. Every stoma different, no one product fits all. No transportation for many. Some homes without running water, bathing facilities. Many lack telephones for follow-up contact.

1.7. Social: Many old people at home with no one to help; women more independent than men, men more dependent on spouses.

1.8. Residence: Referred from all over the state and some surrounding states.

1.9. Psychological: Fear of cancer; devastation by change in body image; inability to express sexual concerns about bodily changes (often not addressed by physicians): female patients not understanding the extent of loss through pelvic exenteration, older black males unable to talk to young white nurses about sexual concerns, patients inadequately prepared preoperatively to aid adjustment to surgical alterations, inability to accept visibility, odors of surgically altered elimination mechanism—ostomy.

1.10. Mental status: Alert preoperative to comatose postoperative.

1.11. General health status: "Sick," nutritional state frequently poor, physical disability of paraplegia and quadriplegia, limitation in range of motion, poor location of stoma for management for some.

1.12. Health conditions treated: 50% to 70% acute and chronic wounds—pressure sores, fistulas, gunshot wounds, pelvic exenteration, necrotizing fasciitis, colostomy and ileostomy, diabetic feet, spina bifida; wounds 20% paraplegics and quadriplegics.

1.13. Health care system factors:

1.13.1. Nurses' caseload: 20 to 30 university hospital inpatients, children's hospital, on call for visits from outpatients, 10 patients in a rural nursing home are seen once a month.

1.13.2. Surgical patients predominantly, some medical.

1.13.3. Average length of stay: 7 days.

1.13.4. Resources:

    1.13.4.1. United Ostomy Association (UOA)—visits, teach patients

    1.13.4.2. Social work referrals for home health, financial assistance

    1.13.4.3. Staff nurses for early referrals

    1.13.4.4. Physician consults

    1.13.4.5. Telephone answering system, pager to receive calls

    1.13.4.6. Office space for record keeping

    1.13.4.7. Computer

2. Foundational capabilities and dispositions

    2.1. Personality, character—internal fortitude has more to do with performance—75% are willing to do, 25% in denial

3. Self-care agency—general capabilities—can do wound/ostomy care unless a physical disability limits, such as paralysis, limited dexterity, visual alteration.

4. Nursing agency

    4.1. Staff nurses—some unit nurses do ostomy care, most do not. Some are quick to identify potential skin problems. All do clean surgical aseptic technique dressings. Consult wound/ostomy nurses for wounds other than clean ones.

    4.2. Wound/ostomy nurses—on call all over hospital, Children's, outpatient.

        4.2.1. Role—assess and treat variety wounds, ostomies, incontinence, use basic pouch—one set up stocked by hospital, must be creative, innovative when standard supplies inadequate to problem; educate patients—video for preoperative ostomy patients, individual teaching and counseling, provide handout instructions for after hospital care and follow-up, seek available resources (UOA, etc.), telephone consult and follow-up on patients three times after hospital discharge.

4.2.2. Time—must travel all over university medical center. If materials needed are not immediately available, must go and find; fistula patients may take from $2\frac{1}{2}$ to 4 hours to do dressings.

4.2.3. Other activities—staff education on ostomy, wound care; committee work—policies and procedures.

4.2.4. Personal education—attend inservice/staff development programs. Need course in diabetic foot care, maintenance of competency for hospital annual checkoff exams.

4.3. Place in organizational structure—directly responsible to _____ as supervisor, and _____ associate administrator for nursing for standards of care.

5. Patient outcomes (therapeutic self-care demand met)

5.1. Upon hospital discharge:

5.1.1. Ostomy patients—changes pouch 1 x day and empties prn; identifies complications that need intervention.

5.1.2. Monitors self and prevention—recognizes signs/symptoms of infection.

5.1.3. Keeps skin clean and dry.

5.1.4. Where there is a massive wound, ileostomy—takes adequate fluids.

5.2. When patient not responsible/able to provide own care (e.g., in denial and unable to deal with the situation), a strong family member must be identified and involved; ostomy nurse, UOA must be contacted for assistance and support.

6. Home requirements: Mirror, running water, bath or shower, stock of pouches/supplies.

7. Finances for supplies, transportation, appropriate bed placement.

Problem Areas

1. Patients: Misuse of emergency room for obtaining supplies.

1.1. 40% are readmitted for complications.

1.2. Most infections are hospital incurred; also pressure sores.

1.3. Lack of clear data on patient outcomes.

1.4. How to empower patients to ascertain that hospital personnel maintain proper technique—gloves, etc., to prevent infection.

2. Physicians: Not up to date on current wound techniques.

2.1. Failure to wear gloves for wound care, do not wash hands—all lead to increased wound infections; suggestions given by nurses to adhere to standards are ignored; at present, no formal way to change MD behavior; failure of some physicians to fully explain the end result meaning of some major procedures' effect on patient's lifestyle, especially sexuality.

2.2. Decision to be made for some patients (especially terminal ones) whether to try to maintain a wound or heal it.

3. Wound/ostomy nurses: Inadequate system to ensure initial contact with patients for preoperative teaching, early identification of problem areas to prevent infection, increasing severity of wounds, lack of time to do preoperative teaching because of day of surgery admissions—teaching makes a definite difference in recovery period re: expectations, complications; not always consulted about patients to prevent or manage problems; no guidelines for when wound/ostomy nurses should be contacted—some patients could be managed by floor nurses; no established effective system for patient follow-up on discharge—need a place for a nurse clinic, possibly at the new community health facility to follow up on these patients; problems with home health follow-up; lack of hospital system to obtain reimbursement for this specialty nurse service; no data to reveal the cost savings to the hospital for the wound/ostomy nurses services; demands on wound/ostomy nurses' time in preceptoring students, for which the hospital is paid $500 per week.

Conclusions

1. At present, there is no organized system for providing this specialty form of health care that would most cost-effectively utilize this service for the benefit of patients and hospital.

2. The wound/ostomy nurses are stretched to cover vast areas and problems and yet are not consulted in some areas that could benefit from their services. Their special knowledge and skills and time could be utilized more effectively and efficiently through planning to help reduce some of the identified problems and their frustrations with them. With a focus on development of a more effective, efficient system for this service, cost savings to the hospital as well as benefits to patients could be achieved.

Goals

1. Patient—effectiveness in increasing healing; prevention of infections; effective management of self/dependent care, achievement of a more effective lifestyle
2. Hospital—increase cost-effectiveness by:
   2.1. Decreasing length of stay
   2.2. Preventing infection (nosocomial)
   2.3. Preventing pressure sores
   2.4. Reducing readmissions

Actions to Meet Goals

1. Develop a system to achieve continuity of care between outpatient and inpatient patient care.
2. Develop critical paths for each type of patient—ostomy, wound care, pressure sores. These might address both nursing practitioners concerning inpatient and outpatient care responsibilities.
3. Develop a documentation system—forms to keep a record of patient outcomes—wound healing, infections, how patient/family manage the needed care, number of readmissions and cause; and follow patient progress on both nursing practitioners, inpatient and outpatient services; also generate for administrative purposes information about nurses' workload—cases seen, time involved, results achieved, also time spent in staff education, committee work, consulting with physicians and others, etc.
4. Develop a method for analysis of the data. Here Dr. _____ of the School of Nursing might be consulted about wound care.

5. Develop guidelines for referral of patients to the wound/ostomy care patients. Make clear what floor nurses should be expected to handle.

6. Commend floor nurses for appropriate early referrals; send note for personnel file for a job well done.

7. Perhaps try to have someone on each unit serve as monitor for impending problems.

8. Provide inservices on the guidelines and findings from collection of data about patient outcomes regarding nosocomial infections, prevention of pressure sores, etc.

9. Seek consultation with nursing administration about how to deal with physician technique problems regarding hospital standards.

10. Investigate financial information about costing out the service, cost savings benefits from reduction in length of stay, and reimbursement of the service. Consult with nursing administration about this.

11. Explore the possibility of setting up a nurse-conducted clinic at the community outpatient facility for follow-up wound/ostomy, diabetic foot care to help reduce emergency room misuse and hospital readmissions.

12. Develop a flowchart for patient contact points in the process of care to identify points of overlap, gaps in care, and what should be attended to at each contact point. Link to critical paths.

13. Explore the possibility for computer tracking of patients for follow-up purposes.

14. Set up a regular weekly planning time to review what has been accomplished, problems to be addressed, and strategies or actions to be taken for them.

15. Submit reports of present meeting to participants for review, correction, additions, and further planning.

16. Submit a summary report to supervisor of patient outcomes and administrative data on a quarterly basis.

17. Establish a time for another meeting of the three participants in this session and any other persons who might be administratively interested and involved.

Second Meeting—2 Months Later

Current Activities

1. Computer program installed for data collection of list of patients by setting—medical, oncology, etc.; diagnosis; client visits; number of visits; wound—size, location, appearance; admission/discharge; lab values; comments—can add data.
2. Prevalence and incidence study—by floor and nurse. Discussed need to get epidemiologist involved, potential for including physicians and other services.
3. One nurse has completed diabetic foot course; the other is to go in next month.

Further Description of Patient Population and Nursing

1. Basic conditioning factors
   1.1 Socioeconomic level seems to have no bearing on management (except for supplies). Lack of money for supplies necessitates nurses having to find possible sources—Ostomy Association, old products from product reps when new ones come out, gifts from product reps and other enterostomal therapists; giving out what is allowable to patient. Problem is, every stoma is different; no standard one fits all. Nurses have to pursue possible sources for supplies or funding of them. Talked about seeking help through social work, civic organizations to sponsor.
2. Self/dependent care agency
   2.1. Personal feelings affect performance of self-care
       2.1.1. Fear
       2.1.2. Repulsion
       2.1.3. Denial—some paraplegics seem to forget the lower body, concentrate on upper body
       2.1.4. Loss of sense of control over life as affected by elimination

2.2. Means and criteria for selecting caregiver (dependent care agent)

    2.2.1. Patient too sick to perform

    2.2.2. Evidence of support network—is a regular visitor

    2.2.3. The person by the bedside the most

    2.2.4. The person patient lives with

    2.2.5. The one who does the most hands-on care

    2.2.6. Observation of personality type—Type A helps; Type B wants to help but concerned about getting in the way; the others do nothing

    2.2.7. Observation of family dynamics—anger, repulsion, etc.

    2.2.8. Facilitating factors:

        2.2.8.1. Love of person evident—relative caring.

        2.2.8.2. Sense of responsibility.

        2.2.8.3. Hopefulness—overcome by working through to the future—get beyond now, together, we can do it.

        2.2.8.4. Belief in self—mentally, emotionally, spiritually—can do.

        2.2.8.5. Knowledge of availability of RN support after discharge—RN gives name, phone number as resource available for any problem, anytime, will call back.

3. Action demands (Therapeutic self-care demand)

    3.1. Change pouch 1 x day.

    3.2. Empty as feel pressure throughout the day; frequency depends on type of surgery.

    3.3. Establish routine—regulation may take from 6 weeks to 3 months; with complications, may take a year.

    3.4. Monitor self for complications, changes; call nurse if change color.

    3.5. Pick and choose what to do.

4. Patient self-care and nursing agency

    4.1. Patient "must own" the wound to do something about it.

4.2. Nursing agency—order of nursing actions:

    4.2.1. Work with feelings.

    4.2.2. Give sense of control.

    4.2.3. Teach procedures as routine for self and self and others.

    4.2.4. Emphasize routine as normal that all have.

    4.2.5. Teach use of alternatives (e.g., bathing—basin, bathroom, travel)

5. Nursing agency—patient approaches

    5.1. Work with feelings first—fear, repulsion, denial, concerns about smell—as normal, but aggravated by change in diet, antibiotics, will become normal.

    5.2. Altered body image, especially young, single—build body image.

    5.3 Grieving process—loss—relate to amputation—scared, normal to deny, be angry.

    5.4. Stimulate patient/family to get excited about it, want to do.

    5.5. Involve in care—"we" help to heal; reward for little things—positive reinforcement, never negative.

    5.6. Draw on related types of experiences—care of a baby, etc.

    5.7. Family feeling of guilt about type of care needed—support, reassure.

    5.8. When acceptance stage begins, start teaching procedures.

    5.9. Work with who you are ("own it").

    5.10. Work with relationships—can train together, if demonstrate anxiety—do separately, when comfortable, do together; sexual concerns—get specific, men not comfortable talking to woman nurse, talk sex as routine; can talk to some partners, others do not listen; talk to one partner separate from the other, then bring together.

    5.11. Women with pelvic exenteration not aware of effects on sexuality; help adjust.

    5.12. Build sense of control—teenagers not go to school without it, fearing reactions of their peers.

5.13. Teach about disease process (e.g., diverticulitis, temporary versus permanent or unknown).

6. Nursing agency and interdisciplinary

6.1. Patient concerns about sexuality in pelvic exenteration—lack of vagina; urge surgeons to build one so patients feel more normal.

6.2. Early involvement with patients makes a difference in outcome.

6.2.1. Stoma markings—prior to surgery, RN measures patient's abdomen in sitting and lying positions, contours of body, etc., to select site for ostomy for best results, fewer complications, better adherence of pouch.

6.2.2. Preoperative notification—time to prepare patient properly about expectations, follow-up. If do above, can reduce problems by 50%.

6.2.3. When patient not handling well, situational versus long-term depression, refer for counseling, antidepressant.

6.2.4. Consult social work, dietary, physical therapy, occupational therapy, home health, etc.

6.2.5. Neuro is multidisciplinary, a support network.

Expense/Revenues (Budget Not Done as Yet;
the Following Are Estimates)

1. Expenses—salaries, office, computer, education, etc.—$120,000 per year gross estimate

2. Use of time

2.1. Nursing practitioner's patient visit—first visit—1½ hours, follow-up visit—45 minutes, see 3 to 4 times during 7-day hospitalization

3. Charges

3.1. Outpatient—15 minutes—$29.00; 30 minutes—$106.00; 1 hour—$212.00.

3.2. Average visit—30 to 45 minutes.

3.3. Supplies charges separate as major or minor.

3.4. General estimate—outpatient—RN—$106 plus $100.00 supplies; one nurse practitioner's patient—$29 plus $30.00 supplies/visit.

4. Proposed nurse clinic for foot/wound care—estimate of time RN available

4.1. One RN full time in hospital 5 days/week.

4.2. One RN in clinic 2 full days/week and 3 days in hospital.

4.3. Total hospital days available—10.

5. Hospital consults per day—6 to 8, minimum 2 to 3; average time 1 hour for wounds, $1\frac{1}{2}$ for ostomy.

6. Other activities

6.1. Old patients' return visits.

6.2. Run for supplies.

6.3. Answer phone messages—document advice.

6.4. Go to radiology to apply a removed pouch.

6.5. Visit nursing home—teaching staff, writing consults.

6.6. Talking to product reps about supplies.

Follow-Up Activities

Explore activities outlined last meeting. Nurses will do a written analysis describing their patients.

Strategies for
Theory-Based Nursing

In the previous chapters, the utility of nursing theory as a component of the mental model of an organization was demonstrated in relation to the structure and processes associated with nursing administration. This chapter is concerned with moving a mental model for nursing from the conceptual stage to the practice arena. Specifically, it describes various strategies for developing the self-care deficit nursing theory in practice and has as its primary focus staff development through various educational approaches. Nurses employed in health care agencies vary extensively in knowledge about formalized nursing theories as well as in education and experience. With such diversity, strategies for relating theory to practice and developing nursing theory based practice must be creative and consistent to bring about desired changes in health care. Incorporation of a nursing theory into daily practice in an organization requires making adjustments in many aspects of the nurses' work life: policies, procedures, documentation systems, standards of care, educational programs, and so on. Introduction of new organizational structures, policies, procedures, or even technologies challenges old beliefs and is accompanied by a demand for changes in philosophy, resources, and practices.

Effecting Change

The techniques of managing change are well documented in the literature (McDonald & Muir, 1996; Pischke-Winn & Minnick, 1996) and include

- Identifying the advantages of the change or innovation
- Identifying the leaders in the organization and ensuring their commitment
- Involving the persons affected by the change/innovation in planning, decision making, and evaluation
- Exploring sources of resistance in the organization and addressing them early
- Communicating—providing for multiple sources of information
- Negotiating
- Developing an implementation plan using tools such as a critical path technique
- Providing appropriate education/training sequenced in a realistic, timely manner
- Providing concise practical guidelines

The application of these techniques to making the mental model of nursing a reality is discussed in later sections of this chapter.

Stevens (1977) commented that continuity and change are two halves of a complementary system. Change is a means to an end. Eventually change should result in a new state of continuity. Also, while the change is occurring, continuity must be addressed, incorporating the change into continuity to prevent chaos. Developing strategic plans to manage change and identifying activities associated with achieving the end goal(s) are important components of the change process. By having a clearly defined end product in mind, there can be flexibility in the processes and activities associated with effecting the desired change. A critical path mapping out the processes and activities may be helpful, especially if appropriate evaluation points are identified and a system is in place for making adjustments based on contingencies that arise. While implementing theory-based nursing practice, there will always be distractions—other priorities, changing allocation of resources, changes in personnel, and so on. As much as possible, changes associated with introduction of theory-based practice should be incorporated into the day-to-day revision activities that are always occurring. For example, if an admission form is to be changed, the utility of the nursing theory in making that form more useful and reflective of the patient variables of concern to nursing should be considered. Standards are constantly being revised. These should be considered in light of the nursing theory. Thus, the changes are systematically and constantly incorporated into the ongoing operation.

Stevens (1977) suggested that activity plans associated with the change should include the following phases:

1. Information on a "need-to-know" basis
2. Education/training for those whose activities will be altered
3. Administrative changes required to support the change
4. Testing the change on a small scale
5. Evaluation of the trial
6. Adaptation based on the trial and related evaluation
7. Diffusion of the change throughout the organization as appropriate

Implementing a Mental Model for Nursing in Delivery of Nursing Services

The Strategic Plan

A strategic plan for implementing a mental model for nursing should be developed in consultation with those to be affected by the change. Development of the plan should address the goals to be achieved, the change process, communication, areas of impact, and evaluation of the process (Allison, 1985; McLaughlin, 1994; Walker, 1993).

■ Objectives/Goals to Be Achieved

Long-range and short-term goals and objectives should be established. Time frames for achievement of the objectives should be specified. Provision should be made for continuing articulation of the implementation process with ongoing activities of the organization. Key people to be involved and affected by the change should be identified. An appropriate committee structure should be specified. Involvement of staff nurses as well as leaders in committee work for developing standards of care and practice, documentation tools or forms, educational programs, and other activities helps nurses learn the theory and attain commitment through knowledge gained from involvement. When such activities are part of committee work, the way we want nursing to be practiced becomes accepted and thus, hopefully, internalized.

■ *The Change Process*

Direction from change theory should be incorporated into the planning process, including accommodating

- ※ Felt need
- ※ Ownership
- ※ Pacing
- ※ Understanding the learning curve
- ※ Information sharing
- ※ Perceptual transformation (Rogers, 1989) and values clarification
- ※ Resistance to change—cultural, social, organizational, psychological

The impact of the introduction of the planned change on individuals, programs, and projects that are currently in progress or planned for in the near future should be explored. Factors that may interfere with or affect the timing of the implementation process should be considered. These should include consideration of recently completed projects and activities currently in process. If staff have recently completed or are currently investing energy into projects with goals that conflict with the planned change, there will be strong resistance to the change. Organizational changes that are planned or are in process should also be considered. Strategies for change associated with each phase of the change process should be identified.

Work redesign is a topic that has received much attention in the literature. For the most part, this involves examining activities that are currently being carried out and setting up some sort of brainstorming activities among the staff to determine how these activities can be modified or assignment of tasks can be adjusted to effect a more efficient operation. Smeltzer and Formella (1996) reported the success of using a survey tool to understand staff values and set the stage for restructuring by opening channels of communication and stimulating discussion. Although these work redesign projects are useful, incorporating attention to the mental model of nursing in such projects provides for addressing the content as well as the context of practice.

Erbin-Roesemann and Simms (1997), in research exploring locus of control, empowerment, and work excitement, found that internal sense of personal control correlated positively with work excitement. People with an internal locus of control tended to be proactive and perceived their jobs to be more enriched, reporting higher levels of job satisfaction. Such people are an asset to instituting change because they are more likely to volunteer in such projects and to seek and share information. Participation in change efforts appears to enhance perceptions of control, with corresponding increased job satisfaction and likelihood of successful redesign outcomes.

■ Communication

Communication includes formal and informal communication, information, and education. "Need-to-know" levels about the change should be identified and appropriate strategies to meet those needs developed. The need may be at the level of information sharing, working knowledge, or in-depth understanding. A specific education program related to the change and maintaining the change should be developed. This should address all components of the organization that are affected by the change, from the orientation of new staff to the end of employment interviews.

Public relations and promotional activities should be part of the strategic plan. These include not only informing top administration and others in the institution or agency but overtly announcing the proposed change through newsletters, posters, presentations, contests, and other means. A variety of means can be used to involve nursing staff and others to promote acceptance of theory-based nursing practice.

■ Evaluation of the Process of Implementation

As identified in previous sections of this book, implementation of theory-based practice and structural, process, and outcome components of the health care enterprise are interactive. The change should affect all of the following, and the nature of the impact should be explored, with appropriate strategies for bringing about desired revisions/modifications identified:

※ Goals, philosophy, standards of nursing practice
※ Description of patient/client populations
※ Clinical decision making, design of patient care, systems of delivery
※ Patient/client classification systems
※ Workload measurement systems
※ Policies and procedures
※ Evaluation of outcomes
※ Research

- Staff development and performance appraisal
- Patient/family education programs

The strategic plan should make provision for a process for evaluating the implementation process, including achievement of objectives. An audit/ monitoring system should be specified in relation to the implementation process and a system established for revising the strategic plan and related activities as required.

Recognition of Need and Selection of a Nursing Theory

Ouellet, Rogers, and Gibson (1989) and Laurie-Shaw and Ives (1988) have detailed the process of selecting a nursing model for practice. Although written some years ago, their suggestions still have merit. Selection and acceptance of a nursing theory as a basis for practice is based on congruence with the nurses' beliefs and values about nursing. Values clarification exercises are useful to help nurses understand their values system. These can be followed by an overview of pertinent nursing theories that are consistent with the values expressed. Having nurses describe their experiences with theories of various kinds can help them to appreciate the value of theory in practice, as can presentations and analysis of current patient situations. These activities frequently result in statements similar to that of an experienced nurse who commented some years ago, "This theory gives me the words to say what I do and know to be nursing" (M. B. Collins, personal communication, n.d.). When staff nurses as well as nurse leaders are both involved in the initial selection process, there is a beginning understanding and commitment to the selected theory that must be further fostered and supported. These nurses frequently become the leaders and mentors for others in learning to use the theory. Theory implementation takes place over time, requiring full administrative support—personally, materially, and budget-wise in terms of time, personnel, and use of resources.

Informing Beyond Nursing

Having decided to proceed with theory as a basis for nursing practice, it is politically advisable for nursing administration to discuss and explain the proposed change, including the reasons for the change and the potential benefits, to those in administration—the board of trustees, top and middle management, medical staff, and leaders in other health care disciplines. Communication is an essential component of any changes being implemented.

Staging the Implementation

An initial decision that must be made is whether to start implementation on a small scale, progressing from a pilot unit to other units or whether to begin agency or institutionwide, expecting all units to introduce and work with the theory. In talking with nurses who have been involved in making the changes associated with instituting theory-based practice, no one procedure seems to be more successful than another. The major contributor to success appears to be the commitment of nursing management to such a change.

The change can be managed through a special project employing a project manager who acts as a facilitator of the change. The change can be managed as a part of the day-to-day activities of current managers. In either case, the use of a consultant familiar with the theory to act as facilitator, interpreter, developer, and educator is recommended unless there is an in-house theory expert who can fulfill this role. All persons involved in the change process and in theory-based practice do not need to have the same in-depth understanding of the theory. If and when the proper structural components are in place, it is like driving a car—the driver does not have to know all of the ins and outs of the mechanics and electronics of getting the car to run.

Some units—for example, a rehabilitation unit, where long-term changes in self-care demands are especially marked—will more readily lend themselves to the change. Patients may be acutely ill, but the situation is more stable and conducive to patient learning. With the rapid turnover and short length of stay in other units, creative planning for teaching and utilizing the theory is required. The advantages of going institutionwide include sending a message to employees that there is a mental model for nursing that is valued and also are economic. An expectation is established that no matter where nurses work, the theory will be the basis for practice. It is more economical to orient and provide formal educational programs for many units than for one small unit. Similarly, documentation forms can be uniform and adaptable without having the cost of an entirely different system for each specialty service area. With a common basis for nursing practice, there is more flexibility in utilization of nursing personnel and transfer of nurses from one unit to another or in utilizing casual or float staff. Merging of patient units, services, or agencies within the larger enterprise is facilitated.

Practicing Nursing From the Perspective of Self-Care Deficit Nursing Theory

During the employment process, applicants should be informed that the self-care deficit nursing theory is the basis for nursing practice and an expectation for all nurses who choose to work in the enterprise. This ensures that they know up front what the expectation is if they accept the position. By the same token, the employer is expected to teach them the theory and help them to grow and develop with it—a career development factor.

Learning to practice nursing from the perspective of a particular nursing theory should take place within the practice arena. In facilitating such practice, educators should recognize the difference between helping experienced nurses change their practices and teaching student nurses. Practicing nurses are interested in how nursing theory can improve the care they provide to their patients/clients, how it can help them solve practice-related problems, and how it can facilitate their day-to-day activities. They do not need to be able to define terms, but they need to be able to use the concepts of the theory.

When nurses are new to an organization using theory-based nursing, introduction to the theory should be gradual. New nurses need time to be socialized into the culture of the organization and to learn the clinical specialty area. Moving from the known to the unknown, they move from what they have known about the specialty to how it is practiced in the current setting, gradually incorporating the theoretical perspective. In the socialization process, they should be exposed to the concepts in direct practice to observe and use the documentation system to the extent that they understand it. When finally they are introduced to the theory in a more formal sense, they readily comprehend the basics essential to practice.

Provision of some reading material about the theory before any formal class sessions gives the nurses some idea about the theory. Preferably, this material should illustrate the application of theory in clinical situations. Discussions about patients and patient situations that draw on the nurses' knowledge and experience should recognize the value of what the nurses know and do and thus be a more comfortable way to begin study of the theory. As nurses relate experiences, the nursing variables and parameters of the theory can be teased out and revealed to them. The nurses can begin to see that theory can provide a systematic way to organize their thinking about what they know and do as nursing. This method demonstrates that theory is not totally foreign and remote because it simply explains and shows various aspects and relationships that the nurse needs to examine and deal with in a systematic logical way to attain nursing goals and results.

Practicing from the perspective of self-care deficit nursing theory means that the focus of nursing is on self-care: what is required, what is facilitating self-care, and what is interfering with self-care. Nursing is necessary because of persons' inability, for health-related reasons, to carry out the quantity and quality of self-care that they require. In other words, the nurse is always determining and reviewing the relationships among self-care, therapeutic self-care demand, and self-care capabilities. In doing this, there is always a need to determine the influencing effects of basic conditioning factors and community variables. An outline for an inservice program related to designing nursing systems for patients with acute renal failure is presented in Appendix 12A.

Case analysis of one or more patient situations is one of the most useful ways of helping nurses to practice from a self-care perspective. Through case analysis, the attention of the nurses can be focused on the variables of concern that have been identified, moving nurses from thinking about nursing action in a particular situation to appreciating all of the factors that patients and families may have to deal with. This approach fosters insights into the meaning and focus of the theory. From a cost savings point of view, anticipating what patients have to know and to do is meaningful not only for designing nursing systems and planning for immediate care but for proposing preventive measures to reduce future costs as well.

Educational Resources

The time and format for teaching classes on self-care deficit nursing theory may vary. It has generally been found beneficial to have concentrated periods of 1 or 2 days away from the daily work situation rather than offering 1 or 2 hours over an extended period of time. In the latter arrangement, nurses tend to forget what they learned in the prior week and are always concerned about what is going on in the work situation that may need tending to on their return. A concentrated period without work responsibilities provides freedom to devote their energies to learning. The results of such planned teaching/learning situations indicate that this is cost-effective.

Most basic nursing programs concentrate on provision of nursing on a one-to-one basis. Helping nurses to think in terms of the population they are serving should be a deliberate focus. The following activity is designed to develop that kind of thinking. When the questions have been answered, nurses should have a fairly comprehensive understanding of what is meant by the term *self-care requisites,* the meaning of conditioning factors in relation to self-care requisites, and impact on self-care agency, and they should have a beginning understanding of how self-care deficit nursing theory gives direction to nursing practice and to the development of standards of practice.

Each ward or unit might begin an in-depth study of self-care requisites including the relationship of self-care requisites to conditioning factors by exploring the following questions:

- Which self-care requisites are particularly significant for patients on their unit?
- What constitutes meeting the self-care requisites for the particular population served?
- What tests, measurements, and criteria will help staff to know if a requisite is being met?
- What factors associated with the unit interfere with meeting those self-care requisites?
- What changes could be implemented to lessen the effect of the above interferences?
- what standards of nursing practice should be in place for the unit in relation to self-care requisites?

Development of a mental picture of self-care agency can begin with the presentation of case studies that illustrate the presence or absence of abilities of knowing, decision making, and acting. Case studies illustrating variation in development and exercise of the power components can be discussed. Related sciences can be explored as topics such as motivation for self-care, an important area for nursing practice, are explored as part of improving nursing practice through the expansion of the nurses' knowledge base.

Classes related to specific nursing technologies should also be organized using self-care deficit nursing theory. For example, if nurses are learning about tube feedings, it should be made explicit that the tube feeding is a way of maintaining a sufficient intake of food. However, other requisites of concern when tube feedings are being used include promotion of normalcy, provision of care related to elimination and excrements, and overcoming factors that interfere with development, to name only a few. Any class related to managing a patient requiring tube feeding should include, in addition to technical information about the procedure, reference to the changes in the self-care demand for these kinds of patients and the effect of tube feeding on the development and exercise of self-care capabilities.

Some people are visual learners. Drawing or using models may help these nurses to see relationships between components of the theory and to describe them in real-world terms. This can be done in discussions using a chalkboard or overhead projector or even slides or videotapes (Vancouver Health Department, 1988). Materials such as these are helpful for review purposes as needed and also can be used to make the initial orientation less time consuming and expensive. When a theory is first introduced in an institution or agency, all nurses must go through an orientation. After this, newly employed nurses need to be oriented, and the number may vary depending on the size of the institution and turnover rate. Self-study materials can be useful, particularly if the numbers of new employees are insufficient for group teaching. New nurses need time to adjust and become familiar and comfortable in their working environment before formal classwork.

Flexibility in approach and allowance of time to learn and assimilate the theory are essential considerations. Timing—knowing when to back off as well as when to push ahead—must be addressed so as not to stress nursing staff but instead to promote learning and acceptance. It takes time for nurses to incorporate changes into their thinking and functioning. Support, patience, and persistence in a constructive flexible approach are essential for acceptance and growth in theory-based practice.

Advanced Theory Work

After about a year, when the nurses have become familiar with the basics of the theory from working with it, to foster further growth and development through deeper understanding of the theory and its relation to nursing practice and research, an advanced course might be offered. A valuable area to be explored is self-care agency—the foundational capabilities and dispositions, power components, and self-care operations—analyzing each in the particular patient population of concern in relation to the types of therapeutic self-care demands that must be dealt with. Another area of study might be the predominant basic conditioning factors that most frequently are present or are most difficult to deal with as they affect self-care agency and therapeutic self-care demand.

Exploration of areas where there are knowledge gaps and exploration of how to articulate other bodies of knowledge to the self-care deficit theory of nursing might be interesting and fruitful. As staff work with the theory, it becomes obvious that there are some gaps in basic knowledge essential for the practice of nursing. One of the deficient areas that surfaces relates to development. Nurses have primarily learned about development from the perspective of psychology and not for nursing purposes. They know about stages of development but have not thought, for example, about how health state articulates with those stages or how self-care practices are influenced by developmental factors.

Not all nurses are interested in or required to attend advanced classes or seminars. This opportunity may be provided for those who seek clinical advancement or managerial positions. They become leaders, experts, who help others through the power of their knowledge as well as their position and personal leadership attributes. They take the lead in designing systems of nursing for patient populations and in developing more effective and efficient nursing technologies and systems for delivery of care. Nurses at the advanced level are expected to present papers relevant to their work at local, regional, and even national conferences and possibly to publish as well. This brings recognition of excellence to their institution or agency as well as a sense of personal accomplishment to them.

Nurses at the advanced level may also wish or be expected to conduct clinical studies to improve nursing practice. For example, as experts in their practice area, knowledgeable about the nursing requirements of the patient population served and the available nursing technologies to meet them, they might develop and test techniques for dealing with or enhancing self-care agency or borrow these from another discipline and validate them from the self-care deficit nursing theory point of view. The opportunities and challenges for finding ways to improve nursing care are limitless but are more meaningful when done from a comprehensive structured theoretical perspective. Such work contributes to the development of nursing knowledge as well as to the personal professional growth of the researcher and to the potential benefit to the organization and profession.

Ensuring Continuity of the Change

In addition to using nursing theory in the clinical information system and standards of practice, it may be useful to develop a "Guide for Nursing Practice" to facilitate moving the mental model from the theoretical to the practical and ensuring continuity of the change. In such a guide, what is meant by using self-care deficit nursing theory to guide nursing practice can be made explicit as the processes the nurse follows when working with patients are specified. Also how to analyze the data that are collected in reference to the patient(s) and the action expected as a result of that analysis can be detailed and illustrated through examples.

The benefits of developing such a guide include

- The nature of nursing practice is made explicit so that all nurses know exactly what is meant by "using self-care deficit nursing theory to guide nursing practice." This guide becomes a reference for the standards of nursing practice.
- Persons developing the guide develop an in-depth understanding of the theory and its relationship to practice.
- Deficiencies in nurse preparation to practice in a manner consistent with the guide become apparent and form the basis of a needs assessment for an inservice education program.
- Discrepancies between the way in which a nurse is expected to practice and the element of a recording system become apparent.
- Discrepancies between the way in which a nurse is expected to practice and the elements identified as components of the performance evaluation standards and criteria become apparent.

The guide for nursing practice should be utilized in the orientation program of new staff. Through its use, new staff nurses can be helped to understand how nursing is to be practiced in the organization.

Summary

Processes and strategies to bring about theory-based practice have been described in this chapter. They have also been described in various publications, many of which contain some of the foregoing strategies. These have been successful to varying extent. A selected list of readings in addition to specific references is included at the end of this chapter. Crucial to any approach to implementing theory-based practice is a firm foundation in understanding of the theory. Each agency must choose the strategies that will work most cost-effectively and efficiently for the particular agency as each goes about making real the mental model for nursing.

References

Allison, S. (1985, June). *Implementation of nursing theory in nursing services*. Paper presented at the Second Annual Institute on Self-Care Deficit Theory of Nursing, Columbia, MO.

Erbin-Roesemann, M. A., & Simms, L. M. (1997). Work locus of control: The intrinsic factor behind empowerment. *Nursing Economics$, 15*, 183-190.

Laurie-Shaw, B., & Ives, S. M. (1988). Implementing Orem's self-care deficit theory. Part I—selecting a framework and planning for implementation. *Canadian Journal of Nursing Administration, 1*(2), 12.

McDonald, V., & Muir, J. (1996, October). Implementing innovations in health care settings. *Canadian Nurse*, pp. 31-33.

McLaughlin, K. (1994). *Strategic planning for theory based nursing practice*. Unpublished paper.

Ouellet, L., Rogers, R., & Gibson, C. (1989). Guidelines for selecting a nursing model for practice. *Canadian Journal of Nursing Administration, 2*(3), 5-9.

Pischke-Winn, K., & Minnick, A. (1996) Project management: Lessons learned from introducing a multitask environmental worker program. *Journal of Nursing Administration, 26*(6), 31-38.

Rogers, M. E. (1989). Creating a climate for the implementation of a nursing conceptual framework. *Journal of Continuing Education in Nursing, 20*(3), 112-116.

Smeltzer, C. J., & Formella, N. M. (1996). Staff surveys: Setting the stage for work restructuring. *Journal of Nursing Quality Care, 11*(1), 6-65.

Stevens, B. J. (1977). Management of continuity and change in nursing. *Journal of Nursing Administration, 27*(4), 26-31.

Vancouver Health Department. (1988). *Teaching self-care deficit nursing theory*. Vancouver, British Columbia: Author.

Walker, D. (1993). A nursing administrator's perspective of use of Orem's self-care deficit nursing theory. In M. Parker (Ed.), *Patterns of nursing theories in practice* (pp. 252-259). New York: National League for Nursing Press.

Additional Suggested Readings

Allison, S. E. (1985). Structuring nursing practice based on Orem's theory of nursing: A nurse administrator's perspective. In J. Riehl-Sisca (Ed.), *The science and art of self-care* (pp. 227-229). Norwalk, CT: Appleton-Century-Crofts.

Allison, S. E., & Nickle, L. (1995). Continuing education for theory based nursing in a service agency. *International Orem Society Newsletter, 3*(1), 5-6.

Duncan, S. (1988, April). Embracing a conceptual model. *Canadian Nurse*, pp. 24-26.

Shea, H., Rogers, M., Ross, E., Tucker, D., Fitch, M., & Smith, I. (1989). Implementing of nursing conceptual models: Observation of a multi-site research team. *Canadian Journal of Nursing Administration, 2*(2), 15-19.

Excerpt From Inservice Program—Nursing System for Patients With Acute Renal Failure

Objectives	Antecedent Knowledge	Related Nursing Knowledge, Skills
Describe the characteristics of acute renal failure. Which requisites will most likely be affected by specific precipitating factors, pathological change, diagnostic studies, physical findings?	Precipitating factors, pathological changes, diagnostic studies, physical findings	

Objectives	Antecedent Knowledge	Related Nursing Knowledge, Skills
Monitor changing health state of patient with acute renal failure— cardiovascular system, urinary system	Diagnostic studies (specific) Prescribed treatment Potential illness trajectory(ies), physical assessment findings	Collecting, storing, transporting specimens (specify) Significance of results and appropriate action Physical assessment—skin, color, edema, respiratory characteristics
Adjust the means of achieving the following depending on the current health state:		
Maintaining a sufficient intake of food and water	Relationship between health state, kidney function, and diet Relationship between health state, kidney function, and fluid intake Sociocultural/religious influences on dietary practices	Food/fluid requirements specific to age, activity, health state, personal preferences, or meeting of other requisites Planning for consumption Specific techniques—e.g., IV Plan for monitoring intake Adjusting intake to changing health state or as required—interpreting significance of clinical behavioral indicators— vital signs, weight changes, fluid retention, change in urinary output, lab results (be specific), pain, etc.
Providing care associated with elimination processes and excrements	Changes that occur in elimination processes associated with acute renal failure—urinary, skin, respiratory, metabolic	Specific care requirements arising from changes in elimination process (e.g., monitoring output, testing urine, skin care)

Objectives	Antecedent Knowledge	Related Nursing Knowledge, Skills
Maintaining a balance between solitude and social interaction and between rest and activity	Relationship between renal function and (a) energy levels, (b) thought processes	Effects of hospitalization/acute illness on relationships and role management
		Management of energy reserves to accomplish personal goals
		Specific techniques for maintaining a balance between rest and activity—(REM sleep)
Preventing hazards to human life: monitoring for impact of hazardous situation, taking appropriate action	Factors hazardous to persons with acute renal failure: infection, smoking, fatigue, stress	Specific techniques for management/control of hazards
Promoting normalcy	Self-concept Relationship between promotion of development and acute, potentially life-threatening illness	Specific techniques for promoting realistic self-concept in presence of acute renal failure (assessment) and for promoting normalcy in presence of acute and potentially life-threatening illness
Bringing about and maintaining living conditions that support life processes and promote development appropriate to developmental stage	Promotion of development specific to various developmental stages	Specific technologies for promoting development for specific developmental stages when this process may be interfered with by hospitalization, acute renal failure
		Overcoming environmental interferences (e.g., hospitalization)

(continued)

Objectives	Antecedent Knowledge	Related Nursing Knowledge, Skills
Assist the patient/family to seek and secure appropriate medical assistance; understand, identify, and work with personal, sociocultural, religious and other values that may affect accessing resources	Medical resources available Methods of accessing those resources Factors that may interfere with accessing resources Specific knowledge and skills patient/family must have to monitor self and take appropriate action in relation to changing health state	Determination of limitations related to knowing, decision making, doing Selection of appropriate methods of helping Determination of nurse role, patient/family role
Be aware of and attend to effects and results of acute renal failure and/or effects or results of treatment of same		

Ensuring the Provision
of Nursing in the Future:
A Summation

In this book, we seek to provide a way to conceptualize nursing and nursing administration as the basis for ensuring the provision of nursing now and in the future. Nurse administrators and nursing practice leaders need mental models through which to think about their work, to structure nursing practice, and to develop ways to ensure that nursing is provided to populations of persons requiring personal assistance with their health care. A definitive comprehensive general theory of nursing such as the self-care deficit nursing theory provides such a model. It speaks to the reality of nursing practice and is simple, yet it reveals the complexities of nursing that need to be explored, studied, and explained. This theory defines the focus and the boundaries of nursing in terms of helping people to manage self and/or dependent care systems—that is, to deal with and overcome actual or potential self-care deficits, enhance, promote, and protect self-care capabilities, and monitor and regulate factors that affect both. The focus of nursing is distinct from that of other health care disciplines, but nursing must be articulated with them to help people reach general goals of life, health, well-being, and effective living. In other words, nursing can be viewed as the medium through which self-care is accomplished and people are helped to maintain and increase their capabilities for self-care. With this focus clear, the limits or boundaries of nursing are known and understood. With this understanding, knowledge developed by other disciplines can be used and/or incorporated into nursing. Overlap and gaps in services between health care disciplines can be seen more clearly. From this perspective, nursing practice and services to patient populations can be structured and developed to meet health care requirements that are appropriate to nursing's domain and complementary to the services and contributions of other health care disciplines, all for the benefit of patients/clients.

The major premise of this book is that the nurse administrator, as the leader for nursing in any nursing organization, big or small, must know and "think" nursing to ensure that nursing is truly provided cost-effectively and efficiently for the benefit of populations served, the profession, the organization, and the community. Nursing administrative leadership is key to making this happen because nurse administrators, at whatever level in the organization, are the ones ultimately responsible for nursing. Nursing leaders in practice and those with designated managerial responsibilities must have a mental model for nursing to structure nursing organizations and their processes if they are to achieve nursing outcomes and be definitively able to say what these are. This means the nurse leader must have a mental model for nursing. The nurse leader, as an advanced nursing practitioner or administrator, must clearly know the nature of the service to be provided and the results to be expected from it. The nurse administrator must be able to conceptualize the dimensions of nursing and have a model for nursing administration. The latter, consistent with self-care deficit nursing theory, addresses the various components or variables of concern in providing nursing for patient populations. The theory provides a guide for structuring nursing practice. The remainder of the book describes what conceptualizations might be put into practice and how, giving practical examples of ways in which to develop administrative processes to ensure the delivery of quality nursing care.

The model for nursing administration mentioned above, found in Figure 3.3, gives direction for development of nursing practice for patient populations, the characteristics of which are described in Chapter 4's Appendix 4A. Particular attention is drawn to the function of design by the nursing professional, a too often neglected function. To date, the notion of design of nursing systems has been given little or no attention in the profession of nursing. A model for design of nursing systems for patient populations is proposed. Figure 6.4 shows the dimensions and conceptualizations of nursing as derived from self-care deficit nursing theory, laid out in flowchart fashion. The factors addressed in this model provide a basis for designing and planning for nursing services for patient populations in relation to general nursing and health goals to be achieved.

A categorization scheme for identifying outcomes of nursing based on the self-care deficit nursing theory is proposed. The categorization model needs to be studied and tested for validity and reliability. But such studies will depend on nurses' practical knowing of the variables in the theory and the development and maintenance of adequate documentation systems. These categories, based on components of the theory, provide a logical, comprehensive framework for evaluating the outcomes of nursing. Figure 10.1 shows the fiscal aspects of nursing administration in relationship to the nursing focus as a basis for examining costs and budgets for nursing, a consideration when looking at nursing productivity in relation to financial outcomes.

When it comes to utilization of nurses, the differences in focus of the basic nurse and the advanced nurse are identified on the basis of a conceptual approach to nursing practice. The nursing theory thus helps to clarify issues related to delivery of nursing services and nursing practice (see Table 11.2). A model (Table 11.3) for delivery of nursing across the continuum of care is proposed. Listed are criteria for decision making about placement of persons in a health care environment on the basis of needs for nursing as defined by the theory. If nursing is the major health service provided by many of these organizations, then the nursing case manager, an advanced nursing practitioner, should play a definitive role in planning and providing nursing across the continuum of care. This nursing role has financial implications and potential for revenue generation for nursing as well.

Finally, the book suggests some strategies for implementing practice from a particular perspective or mental model in an organization. Because nurses employed in an organization may or may not have any knowledge of the particular mental model for nursing that has been adopted by the organization as the basis for practice, it is incumbent on the organization to ensure that these nurses learn the theoretical basis for nursing practice, work from that perspective, and communicate it orally and in written documentation. This ensures commonality of purpose and consistency in practice and communication about patients/clients.

At this stage of development in professional nursing, when no one conceptual framework or mental model for nursing is commonly accepted, valid and reliable nursing theories must be tested in the reality of the nursing work world. The nurse administrator ultimately is the one to promote and support the establishment of a theoretical perspective for nursing practice and must substantiate its effectiveness or ineffectiveness in terms of the purposes and goals of the organization providing the service and the populations being served. Evidence of productivity and effectiveness in results from theory-based nursing, when shared with others through demonstration and publication, can bring about a change in how nursing is practiced in the future. This book proposes an approach to that future and places the responsibility on nursing administration, aided by advanced nursing practitioners, to make that future happen.

Index

About the Authors

Sarah E. Allison, RN, MSN, EdD, was a member of the Nursing Development Conference Group, which did pioneer work in the development of self-care deficit nursing theory. She has been involved as a nursing administrator in the integration of nursing theory and nursing administration for more than 30 years. She is frequently sought out as a consultant and speaker on this topic at national and international nursing conferences and has taught nursing theory at several university schools of nursing. She was formerly Vice President of the International Orem Society and Vice President of Nursing Administration at the Mississippi Methodist Rehabilitation Hospital and Center in Jackson, Mississippi. Her recent publications include "Nursing Theory: A Tool to Put Nursing Back Into Nursing Administration" (with Kathie McLaughlin and Dale Walker) in *Nursing Administration Quarterly* (1991), "Historical Development of the Self-Care Deficit Nursing Theory in Education Practice" in the *International Orem Society Newsletter* (1993), and "Continuing Education for Theory-Based Nursing in a Service Agency" (with Lynne Nickle) in the *International Orem Society Newsletter* (1995).

Katherine E. McLaughlin-Renpenning, RN, MScN, has had experience as a nursing educator as well as a nursing administrator. She has provided consultation services relating to the use of nursing theory to provide direction for nursing practice, education, research, and administration over the past 15 years in Canada and internationally. She is currently President and Chief Nursing Consultant of MCL Educational Services, Inc., and McLaughlin Associates. She has been involved in the development of computer applications using nursing theory as a component of the information-processing model. She is a member of the Self-Care Deficit Nursing Theory Study Group and the Editor of the *International Orem Society Newsletter.* She has also been a speaker nationally and internationally. Recent publications include coauthorship of "The Practice of Nursing in Multiperson Situations, Family and Community" in D. E. Orem's *Nursing: Concepts of Practice* (5th ed.) and authorship of "Implementing Self-Care Deficit Nursing Theory: A Process of Staff Development" in Marilyn Parker's *Patterns of Nursing Theories in Practice,* as well as coauthorship of several articles on computer applications and nursing theory.